Certified Coding Specialist (CCS) Exam Preparation

Fourth Edition

Jennifer Hornung Garvin,
PhD, MBA, RHIA, CPHQ, CCS, CTR, FAHIMA

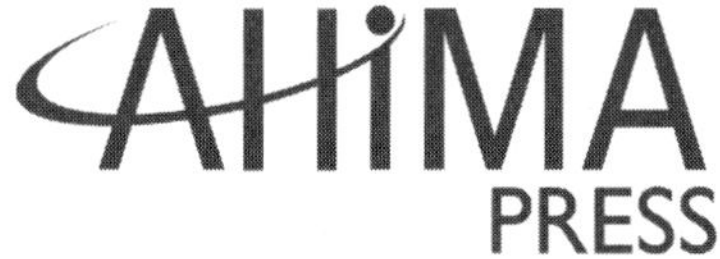

ISBN 978-1-58426-313-5
AHIMA Product No. AC400411

AHIMA Staff:
Kathryn A. DeVault, RHIA, CCS, CCS-P, Technical Review
Katherine Greenock, MS, Editorial and Production Coordinator
Ashley Sullivan, Assistant Editor
Pamela Woolf, Senior Developmental Editor
Ken Zielske, Director of Publications

For more information, including updates, about AHIMA Press publications, visit http://www.ahima.org/publications/updates.aspx

American Health Information Management Association
233 North Michigan Avenue, 21st Floor
Chicago, Illinois 60601-5809
ahima.org

Contents

On the CD-ROM

About the Author

Jennifer Hornung Garvin, PhD, MBA RHIA, CPHQ, CCS, CTR, FAHIMA is currently a Core Research Investigator at the Salt Lake City VA IDEAS Research Center and an Assistant Professor at the University of Utah School of Medicine in the Division of Epidemiology. She is a health information management (HIM) professional with 27 years of experience in HIM and applied informatics. She received an associate of science and a post-baccalaureate certificate in HIM from Gwynedd-Mercy College, bachelor and doctoral degrees from Temple University, a master's degree in business (MBA) from St. Joseph's University, and a graduate certificate in Biomedical Informatics from the Oregon Health and Science University. Her professional training includes a postdoctoral fellow at the Center for Health Equity Research and Promotion (CHERP) sponsored by the Department of Veteran Affairs (VA) at the Philadelphia VA Medical Center (PVAMC) in association with the University of Pennsylvania School of Medicine (SOM).

She was the program director of AHIMA accredited associate and bachelor degrees as well as an AHIMA approved coding certificate program at Gwynedd-Mercy College for nine years before seeking research training. Dr. Garvin served on the AHIMA Board of Directors, as chair of the Research Committee, and as president of Pennsylvania Health Information Management Association (PHIMA) and is currently the president-elect of the Utah Health Information Management Association

Acknowledgments

The author wishes to thank the following individuals for being editors, reviewers, and publishers of previous editions of the *CCS Exam Success Review Book:*

Elizabeth Layman, PhD, RHIA, CCS, FAHIMA
Kathy Arner, LPN, RHIT, CCS, CPC
Genevive Badroe
Christine Staropoli, MS, RHIA, CCS
Angela Picard Carney, PhD, RHIA
Stephen Weiner, DO
Julian Wade Farrior, PhD
Pam Farrior, RPh
Aileen Stanton, CHCO, CCS, CCP
Pauline Graham, RHIT, CHCO, CCS, CCP
Becky Thorson, RHIT, CCS
Linda Donahue, RHIT, CCS, CCS-P, CPC
Christina Benjamin, MA, RHIA, CCS, CCS–P
Dasantila Sherifi, MBA, RHIA

And any other reviewers from past editions who were inadvertently not named.

In addition a special thank you goes to all the HIM professionals who have sent me questions and suggestions regarding the contents of this book. You have made this work extra special.

I also so much appreciate the helpful AHIMA publication staff members who have assisted the production of this text.

About the CCS Exam

Coding professionals who pass the certified coding specialist (CCS) exam are professionals skilled in classifying medical data from patient records, generally in the hospital setting. These coding practitioners review patients' records and assign numeric codes for each diagnosis and procedure. To perform this task, they must possess expertise in the ICD-9-CM and CPT coding systems. In addition, the CCS is knowledgeable of medical terminology, disease processes, and pharmacology. Hospitals or medical providers report coded data to insurance companies, or to the government in the case of Medicare and Medicaid recipients, for reimbursement of expenses. Researchers and public health officials also use coded medical data to monitor patterns and explore new interventions. Coding accuracy is thus highly important to healthcare organizations because of its impact on revenues and describing health outcomes, and in fact, certification is becoming an implicit industry standard. Accordingly, the CCS credential demonstrates tested data quality and integrity skills in a coding practitioner. The CCS certification exam assesses mastery proficiency in coding rather than entry-level skills. Professionals experienced in coding inpatient and outpatient records should consider obtaining this certification. For exam eligibility requirements, visit ahima.org/certification.

Exam Competency Statements

The CCS certification exam is based on an explicit set of competencies. These competencies were determined by job analysis surveys of hospital-based coders. The competencies are subdivided into domains and tasks, as listed here. The CCS exam tests only content pertaining to the following competencies.

Domain 1: Health Information Documentation (15%)

1. Interpret health record documentation using knowledge of anatomy, physiology, clinical disease processes, pharmacology, and medical terminology to identify codeable diagnoses and/or procedures.
2. Determine when additional clinical documentation is needed to assign the diagnosis and/or procedure code(s).
3. Consult with physicians and other healthcare providers to obtain further clinical documentation to assist with code assignment.
4. Consult reference materials to facilitate code assignment.
5. Identify patient encounter type.
6. Identify and post charges for healthcare services based on documentation.

Domain 2: Diagnosis Coding (20%)

1. Select the diagnoses that require coding according to current coding and reporting requirements for acute care (inpatient) services.
2. Select the diagnoses that require coding according to current coding and reporting requirements for outpatient services.

3. Interpret conventions, formats, instructional notations, tables and definitions of the classification system to select diagnoses, conditions, problems or other reasons for the encounter that require coding.
4. Sequence diagnoses and other reasons for encounter according to notations and conventions of the classification system and standard data set definitions such as Uniform Hospital Discharge Data Set (UHDDS).
5. Apply the Official ICD-9-CM Coding Guidelines.

Domain 3: Procedure Coding (20%)

1. Select the procedures that require coding according to current coding and reporting requirements for acute care (inpatient) services.
2. Select the procedures that require coding according to current coding and reporting requirements for outpatient services.
3. Interpret conventions, formats, instructional notations, and definitions of the classification system and/or nomenclature to select procedures/services that require coding.
4. Sequence procedures according to notations and conventions of the classification system/nomenclature and standard data set definitions such as UHDDS.
5. Apply the Official ICD-9-CM Coding Guidelines.
6. Apply the official CPT/HCPCS Level II coding guidelines.

Domain 4: Regulatory Guidelines and Reporting Requirements for Acute-Care (Inpatient) Service (10%)

1. Select the principal diagnosis, principal procedure, complications, comorbid conditions, other diagnoses and procedures that require coding according to UHDDS definitions and *Coding Clinic* for *ICD-9-CM.*
2. Evaluate the impact of code selection on diagnosis-related group (DRG) assignment.
3. Verify DRG assignment based on inpatient prospective payment system (IPPS) definitions.
4. Assign the appropriate discharge disposition.

Domain: 5: Regulatory Guidelines and Reporting Requirements for Outpatient (Ambulatory) Services (10%)

1. Select the reason for encounter, pertinent secondary conditions, primary procedure, and other procedures that require coding according to UHDDS definitions, *CPT Assistant,* and *Coding Clinics* for *ICD-9-CM,* and HCPCS.
2. Apply outpatient prospective payment system (OPPS) reporting requirements:
    - Modifiers
    - CPT/HCPCS Level II
    - Medical necessity
    - Evaluation and Management code assignment (facility reporting)

Domain 6: Data Quality and Management (8%)

1. Assess the quality of coded data.
2. Educate healthcare providers regarding reimbursement methodologies, documentation rules and regulations related to coding.
3. Analyze health record documentation for quality and completeness of coding.
4. Review the accuracy of abstracted data elements for data base integrity and claims processing.
5. Review and resolve coding edits such as Correct Coding Initiative (CCI), Medicare Code Editor (MCE), and Outpatient Code Editor (OCE).

Domain 7: Information and Communication Technologies (5%)

1. Use computer to ensure data collection, storage, analysis, and reporting of information.
2. Use common software applications (for example word processing, spreadsheets, email, etc.) in the execution of work processes.
3. Use specialized software in the completion of HIM processes.

Domain 8: Privacy, Confidentiality, Legal, and Ethical Issues (6%)

1. Apply policies and procedures for access and disclosure of personal health information.
2. Apply AHIMA Code of Ethics and the Standards of Ethical Coding.
3. Recognize/report privacy issues/problems.
4. Protect data integrity and validity using software or hardware technology.

Domain 9: Compliance (6%)

1. Participate in the development of institutional coding policies to ensure compliance with official coding rules and guidelines.
2. Evaluate the accuracy and completeness of the patient record as defined by organizational policy and external regulations and standards.
3. Monitor compliance with organization-wide health record documentation and coding guidelines.
4. Recognize/report compliance concerns/findings.

Exam Specifications

The 2011 CCS certification exam has been redesigned for 2011 and consists of the following:

Theory (40% of the exam)—Excludes coding domains 2 and 3

- 60 four-option multiple choice items

Application (60% of the exam)—Domains 2 and 3 and coding health records

- 21 multiple choice items
- 8 multiple select items
- 56 quantifiable fill-in-the-blank items—coding medical record cases

The total testing time for the CCS exam is 4 hours. Be sure to pace yourself during the exam and use your time wisely.

Instructions and official guidelines for coding medical records are included in the following resources: ICD-9-CM, CPT, UHDDS, *Coding Clinic for ICD-9-CM,* and *CPT Assistant.* However, hospitals and other organizations may develop their own procedures in the absence of approved guidelines. To ensure consistent coding, the specific coding instructions have been developed for use during the CCS exam. The exam coding instructions do not supersede or replace official coding advice and guidelines included in the recommended exam study resources (ahima.org/certification). *For CCS exam coding instructions, see pages 14–16 in the Introduction of this book.*

The Commission on Certification for Health Informatics and Information Management (CCHIIM) manages and sets the strategic direction for the certifications. Pearson Vue is the exclusive provider of AHIMA certification exams. To see sample questions and images of the new exam format, visit ahima.org/certification.

What Books to Bring

Beginning **July 7, 2011,** candidates must bring the 2011 versions of *ICD-9-CM Volumes 1 through 3* CPT, and the American Medical Association CPT codebook. (Only the AMA codebook is permitted.) A medical dictionary is optional.

Candidates without the required codebooks will not be permitted to test and will forfeit their application fee. Candidates who do not bring all the required books, or whose books do not have the correct year, will not be allowed to test. For the most up-to-date exam information visit ahima.org/certification.

How to Use This Book

The CCS practice questions and practice exams in this book test knowledge of content pertaining to the CCS competencies published by AHIMA and available at ahima.org/certification. The multiple choice practice questions and practice medical cases along with two practice exams are presented in a similar format to what might be found on the CCS exam.

This book contains 60 practice multiple choice questions and five practice case studies along with two practice exams, each with 60 multiple choice questions and 13 cases studies. (Additional coding exercises can also be found in the Introduction of this book.) Each multiple choice question is identified with one of the nine CCS domains, so you will be able to determine whether you need knowledge or skill building in particular areas of the exam domains. Most answers include rationales and references for further guidance. Pursuing these references will help you build your knowledge and skills in specific domains.

To most effectively use this book, work through all of the practice questions first. This will help you identify areas in which you may need further preparation. For the questions that you answer incorrectly, read the associated references to help refresh your knowledge. After going through the practice questions, take one of the practice exams. Again, for the questions that you answer incorrectly, refresh your knowledge by reading the associated references and study resources listed in the back of this book.

About the CD-ROM

The CD-ROM accompanying this book contains 180 practice multiple choice items covering all nine CCS domains. The self-scoring multiple choice questions on the CD can be set to be presented in random order, or you may choose to go through the questions in sequential order by domain. You may also choose to practice or test your skills on specific domains. For example, if you would like to build your skills in domain 3, you may choose only domain 3 multiple choice questions for a given practice session.

To install the practice exams on your computer, follow these steps:

1. Insert the CD-ROM in your computer's CD/DVD drive.
2. Double-click the .exe file.
3. When asked if you would like to extract files from this archive, select Yes.
4. Read and accept the license agreement.
5. If offered an installation path, choose the default path suggested.
6. A message will appear stating that the files have been successfully extracted.
7. The Setup Wizard will open.
8. Follow on-screen instructions through setup and installation.

Minimum system requirements: Intel Pentium II 450MHz or faster processor (or equivalent) with 128MB of RAM running Microsoft Windows 2000, XP, Vista, or Windows 7. The CD software is written for a Microsoft Windows environment. To run the test simulations on a Macintosh, you will need to simulate a Windows environment using additional software for a Mac, such as Apple's Bootcamp. AHIMA cannot guarantee this CD will run on a Mac. This software product is designed to work on Windows 2000, XP, Vista, and Windows 7.

Under most circumstances, installation will be easy. *Important: If you have problems with installation, open the Read Me file on the CD-ROM for detailed help instructions.*

Introduction

The purpose of this book is to provide practice exercises for the certified coding specialist (CCS) exam through a review of important ICD-9-CM and CPT coding material. Two simulations of the CCS exam are included in this book to help you to improve test performance within the context of the four-hour exam. The content of this book is not intended to predict what will be on the CCS exam, and utilizing *CCS Exam Preparation* does not guarantee a passing score. However, *CCS Exam Preparation* does provide a focused method of preparing for the exam through review, practice, and exam simulation.

Steps for Success

1. Review basic coding principals in coding books and then test yourself via the exercises provided in this book and on the accompanying CD.
2. Review relevant American Hospital Association *Coding Clinic* articles. Read as many issues of the *Coding Clinic* as possible but be sure to review the most recent five years (2006 through 2010) beginning with the most recent articles. As noted, the *Coding Clinic* articles used to develop the 2011 CCS exam end with the fourth quarter of 2010. Knowledge of *Coding Clinic* is crucial for success on the CCS exam. Also be sure to review the most recent ICD-9-CM Official Guidelines for Coding and Reporting, which are included in *Coding Clinic*. The national standards for coding practice are provided in *Coding Clinic* and it is therefore the basis for establishing the correct answers related to ICD-9-CM on the CCS exam.
3. Review a CPT educational text and complete exercises for areas in which more skill is needed. Review the guidelines section of each section of the CPT codebook to ensure adequate knowledge of the details of each area.
4. Review the American Medical Association *CPT Assistant* from the most recent issues going backward as far as possible.
5. Complete the introductory exercises and practice questions in this book.
6. To prepare psychologically for the experience of taking the four-hour CCS exam, simulate the experience by completing a practice exam *in one sitting.*

   Along with practice questions and case studies, this book contains two practice exams (each with 60 multiple choice questions and 13 cases studies) and additional coding exercises, which appear at the end of this Introduction.

   The CD contains three sets of 60 multiple choice practice questions, which can be presented in sequential order (by domain) or random order for a more challenging experience.
7. Follow up with the references and other CCS study resources. Ask CCS-credentialed professionals for clarification on items that are unclear.

For more information on the exam, refer to the About the CCS Exam section earlier in this book or visit ahima.org/certification.

Make Plans for CCS Success

In order to develop a good plan of study, it is important to reflect on what you have read so far. Use a calendar to determine how much time you have to prepare.

- How many hours can you spend per week studying?
- How many weeks do you have to study before the exam? (Exclude weeks when you have personal or family events.)

Good preparation using the steps to success can help you achieve a successful exam experience!

Self-Evaluation Notes

Each person who studies for the CCS exam has a different skill set. One of the goals for using this book is to determine your areas of weakness. Strategies can then be developed to make weak areas stronger. Take a few minutes to complete this self-evaluation so that your specific needs can be addressed. Use this self-evaluation to help gather resources before working through the remainder of this book.

I need more practice in these areas:

1. ______________________________
2. ______________________________
3. ______________________________

I can strengthen these areas by:

1. ______________________________
2. ______________________________
3. ______________________________

I need these resources to help me:

1. ______________________________
2. ______________________________
3. ______________________________

Coding Challenges

The following is an outline of potentially challenging coding issues. When possible, obtain the reference materials listed in the back of this book and utilize them. Creating a study schedule and reviewing materials that address your weaknesses will enable you to achieve your goals. Many people find that meeting with a small study group each week in person can help you stay on track. In addition to study group support, there is an AHIMA Community of Practice (CoP), Studying for the CCS, which provides online assistance and resources for members. As you review the different areas of content, identify any weaknesses that you need to focus on for improvement.

In order to do well on the multiple choice section of this book, reference material related to the exam content should be memorized. It is not possible to memorize everything, so developing a study strategy is important. Be sure to read the About the CCS Exam section earlier in this book to fully understand the exam contents and what should be coded in the medical cases. Determine weak areas and study to improve those areas. Focus on clinical scenarios and reimbursement topics that would apply to the "average" hospital.

Codebooks are allowed during the CCS exam. Refer to the AHIMA Certification website (ahima.org/certification) for a current list of allowable codebooks. Furthermore, materials in codebooks must be permanently affixed inside your codebooks. Remember too that you will need to gain speed using the codebooks because an encoder is not used to assign codes during the exam. In order to hone this skill, practice coding exercises by timing yourself to evaluate your speed and accuracy using actual codebooks.

The following are highlights to remember:

- Because national coding guidelines and references are used for the CCS exam, evaluate your hospital guidelines to identify any difference between the two. Be sure to code according to national guidelines.
- Recent issues addressed in *Coding Clinic* and CPT Assistant are important. Begin your review from the most recent to the oldest issues. Identify areas that are confusing or have been revised over time. Make sure you understand the most recent decisions regarding any particular coding issue.
- Knowledge of MS-DRGs and APCs are important. Which MS-DRGs will be affected by major comorbidities or complications (MCCs) and complications or comorbidities (CCs) is key information. You should have a general idea about common MS-DRGs for the average hospital in the United States and the reimbursement methodology of APCs. For example, what status indicators mean and how to assign evaluation and management (E/M) levels if given a template.
- An understanding of accurate principal diagnosis assignment is key. It is essential to know the disease processes that underlie ethical coding. Much of this knowledge is based in *Coding Clinic* reference material and the Uniform Hospital Discharge Data Set (UHDDS).
- Generally, cases on the exam reflect common cases that a coder in an average hospital would code. Determine if you have a knowledge deficit in any common coding areas because your facility does not treat that type of patient. For example, some facilities do not provide services for newborns, deliveries, heart catheterizations, coronary artery bypass grafts (CABGs), or neonatal intensive care. If you work in such a facility, you will need to strategize how to gather expertise in these areas. One way to gain expertise is to review the coding exercises in a basic coding book and to use an encoder to determine the MS-DRGs associated with the exercises.
- On the CCS exam, national coding principles are emphasized. Reviewing of the last two years of the Journal of AHIMA is a worthwhile endeavor. Be mindful of such topics as future nomenclatures such as ICD-10 and the Health Insurance Portability and Accountability Act (HIPAA). Also, keep in mind that sometimes coders get into habits that may subtly deviate from coding guidelines. Be on alert and identify any of these habits in order to correct them.

ICD-9-CM Review

The following is an outline of some of the more important areas to know.

Infectious Disease

- Review the most recent guidelines regarding sepsis (038.x + SIRS code) versus septicemia (038.x). They require that a code from 038 be used followed by 995.91. If septic shock is also documented, 995.92 and 785.52 should be assigned.

Diabetes

- Review the definition of fifth digits in this category.
- Understand the difference between type I and type II diabetes and the pathophysiology of both types.

Respiratory

- Remember to use the code for the specific type of pneumonia if the cause of the pneumonia is documented in the medical record by the provider.
- Know the criteria for recognizing gram-negative and other specific types of pneumonia when documented in the medical record.
- Review the various types of chronic obstructive pulmonary disease (COPD) and how the acute exacerbation of each is coded. Know the criteria for coding asthma with status asthmaticus as specified in *Coding Clinic* and code only when documented in the record.
- Review the criteria for coding respiratory failure and when it may be sequenced first.

Procedures

- Understand how procedures, sometimes performed at the patient's bedside, affect the MS-DRG assignment. Some examples are transbronchial biopsies, ventilator usage, excisional debridement, and tracheostomies.
- Be careful to assign debridement codes appropriately. Do not code an excisional debridement unless there is documentation in the record reflecting that an excisional debridement was performed. Review the *Coding Clinic* guidance associated with excisional debridement.

Gastrointestinal

- Use a combination code whenever available that incorporates a hemorrhage and the specific disorder. Use the 578.x category as an additional code when no combination code has been created or when the cause of the hemorrhage is unknown.
- Understand the difference between a direct (no path report) versus an indirect hernia (path report will show a hernia sac) and how to code them.

Delivery and Pregnancy

- Understand the definition of fifth digits and when to use them. Remember that the fifth digit of "4" is only used for a postpartum complication not in the same episode of the delivery. If you work at a facility that does not perform deliveries, use the review exercises in another coding text to improve your knowledge in this area.
- Memorize the definition of a normal delivery and know the parameters for using the 650 code.

- Recognize that, at a minimum, delivery charts must have the following types of codes: delivery diagnosis code (6xx code), outcome of delivery (V2x.xx), and procedure code (73.59 if no other procedure performed).
- Remember that medical conditions associated with pregnancy, delivery, and puerperium require both a 6xx code as well as a disease code. For example, postpartum anemia is coded as 648.22 and 285.9.

Ectopic Pregnancy and Miscarriages

- Understand the definition of fifth digits and when to use them.
- Understand how to code complications of ectopic pregnancy and abortions during the admission for treatment of the ectopic pregnancy or abortion. Review the Inclusion notes for 639.x category in the ICD Tabular Index and know when to use them.

Anemia

- Review the anemia coding. In particular, there are anemia codes for anemia in chronic illness. Also, blood loss anemia is a commonly associated condition with chronic bleeding and acute bleeding. Be sure to know when to code acute versus chronic blood loss anemia. It is also important to review national guidelines regarding postoperative anemia.

Cardiovascular Conditions

- Remember to specify the location of the myocardial infarction and any comorbidities that will affect the DRG assignment such as arrhythmias, heart failure, hypotension, and so on.
- Review and understand sequencing issues pertaining to arteriosclerotic heart disease (AHD) and unstable angina in *Coding Clinic*.
- Review the coding of cerebral infarctions and sequelae such as aphasia and hemiplegia.
- Review coding cardiac procedures such as cardiac catheterizations and bypass surgery. If you do not have exposure to this type of chart, practice coding these issues using a coding exercise book.

Neoplasms

- Review the definitions of the categories in the table.
    - The primary site is where the cancer arises.
    - A secondary neoplasm is present whenever the neoplasm leaves the organ of origin (where it began). This can occur when the neoplasm travels through the blood and/or the lymphatic system or via direct growth (direct extension) into another adjacent tissue.
- Remember that looking up the morphology type can lead you to the primary site (for example, renal cell carcinoma arises in the kidney).
- Review the suggested steps in *ICD-9-CM Coding Handbook with Answers,* which are synopsized as follows:
    - Look up the morphology and code the primary site if given.
    - If no primary site code is indicated by the morphology type, the neoplasm table must be used.
    - If the term "metastatic" is used ambiguously, assume the following are secondary sites: bone, brain, diaphragm, heart, liver, lymph nodes, mediastium, meninges, peritoneum, pleura, retroperitoneum, spinal cord, and sites from the 195 category.

Injuries and Burns

- Review the difference between traumatic versus pathological fractures.
- Make sure the most extensive wound is coded and all injured internal organs are coded.
- Review the fifth digits related to intracranial injury, and make sure the appropriate code is used.
- Remember that if burns are located in the same body area, use only the degree of greatest severity. For example, if there are second- and third-degree burns of the forearm, only the third-degree burn of the forearm is coded.

Drugs

- Review the difference between abuse and addiction and the fifth digits associated with them. Also review the coding of procedures associated with this area.
- Review the definition of adverse effect. The following terms indicate an adverse effect of a drug:
  - Allergic reaction
  - Cumulative effect
  - Hypersensitivity
  - Idiosyncratic reaction
  - Paradoxical reaction
  - Synergistic
- Review the definition of poisoning. The following are classified as poisonings when:
  - The drug is administered, taken, or prescribed incorrectly, for example, if an overdose of medication occurs
  - Alcohol is used in conjunction with a drug
  - Street drugs are taken resulting in an overdose or taken in addition to prescribed or over-the-counter (OTC) drugs
  - OTC drugs are taken with prescriptions
  - Two OTC drugs are used together

Complications

- Review this section of the ICD-9-CM codebook to refresh your memory about how these codes are found. Review the Alphabetic and Tabular Indices and what is contained within each category.
- The best way to review this area is to go through the Tabular Index.
- The first area in the Tabular Index contains the three major groupings associated with devices and complications (in the Complications chapter):
  - Mechanical Complications (996.0–996.59)
  - Infection/Inflammation Due to Devices (996.6–996.69)
  - Other Complications (996.7–996.79)
- Review the general complications in the 997 and 998 categories. Remember that a second code is required because of the directions given under the main heading of 997. If the code is not specific to the exact type of complication, a second code should also be used with 998 to denote the specific manifestation. For example, if a patient has intraoperative atrial fibrillation, use 997.1 and 427.31; and if a patient has postoperative septicemia, use 998.59 and 038.9.

- Review the 999 category. Issues such as phlebitis due to IV are listed.
- Complications that occur only in specific body sites are classified in the respective chapter of an ICD-9-CM codebook. For example, postoperative pulmonary embolism (415.11) is found in Chapter 7, Diseases of Circulatory System (390–459). Complications of abortion, pregnancy, labor, or delivery are classified to chapter 11, Complications of Pregnancy, Childbirth, and the Puerperium (630–679).

Perinatal Conditions

- Use the V code (V3x.xx) as principal when the admission is for the birth of the infant. Do not use V3x.xx if the admission is not for birth (for example, the patient is transferred).
- Code other perinatal conditions as appropriate such as birth trauma, prematurity, jaundice when documented in the record.

MS-DRGs and Case Mix

Obtain the MS-DRG list for fiscal year 2011(refer to the References section in this book). Highlight the most common MS-DRGs that will occur in the average hospital and look at how they are ordered. This type of study will help you become familiar with the most common MS-DRGs and see the hierarchy of MS-DRG decision trees. Generally, the MS-DRG grouper considers the following information: whether the patient had a procedure, the age of the patient, and whether there was a major comorbid condition (MCC).

It is important to review the definitions of case mix and case-mix index (AHIMA 2010, 40–41).

- Case mix: 1.) A description of a patient population based on any number of specific characteristics, including age, gender, type of insurance, diagnosis, risk factors, treatment received, and resources used 2.) Set of categories of patients (type and volume) treated by a healthcare organization and representing the complexity of the organizations case load.
- Case-mix index (CMI): The average relative weight of all cases treated at a given facility or by a given physician, which reflects the resource intensity or clinical severity of a specific group in relation to the other groups in the classification system; calculated by dividing the sum of the weights of diagnosis-related groups for patients discharged during a given period divided by the total number of patients discharged.

If you do not code inpatient records on a routine basis, it is important to obtain a list of MS-DRGs from the Centers for Medicare and Medicaid Services (CMS 2011, search for *DRG relative weights*). If possible, put some of the exercises or cases in this book into the MS-DRG grouper to familiarize yourself with common MS-DRGs. Switch the principal diagnosis and note how the MS-DRG changes. Also note which MS-DRGs are affected by MCCs.

Review the MS-DRG weights of the most common MS-DRGs that would occur in an average hospital in the United States. The following is a list, which is by no means all-inclusive, of some common clinical scenarios that might form the basis of further study.

Pneumonia
Congestive Heart Failure
Cholecystitis and Cholecystectomy
Malignant Neoplasms with Associated Treatments
    Lung
    Breast
    Prostate
    Colon

- Fracture of Femur with Associated Treatments
    - Total Hip Replacement
    - Open Reduction with Internal Fixation
- Septicemia
- Gastrointestinal Hemorrhage
- COPD with Exacerbation
- Respiratory Failure
- Deliveries
- Newborns
- Anemia

Review the common MS-DRGs that cannot be optimized unless a procedure is found or the principal diagnosis is changed. Try to find some examples.

Use a grouper that you have access to in your work or academic institution or use a free DRG grouper (for example, from irp.com). *Disclaimer: This software application may contain errors and is not endorsed or developed by the author or AHIMA.*

Case-mix Exercises

The following exercises are meant to help you learn more about case-mix analysis and increase your knowledge of MS-DRGs. In actual coding practice, it would only be appropriate to switch the principal diagnoses if the clinical information conformed to UHDDS guidelines that supported a change in principal diagnosis. Try the following exercises. The discharge disposition is discharged to home.

1. A 22-month-old child has pyelonephritis (590.80) and dehydration (276.51) and both are equally treated. Which MS-DRG will have the highest weight?

2. If a 65-year-old patient has pneumonia (486) and congestive heart failure (428.0), which DRG will have a higher weight?

3. If a 70-year-old patient has pneumonia due to *Escherichia coli* (482.82) and an acute exacerbation of COPD (491.21), which DRG will have a higher weight?

4. Case mix (CM) and case-mix index (CMI) calculations: The CM is all of the weights added together. The CMI is the average weight of all the cases in a given dataset or period of time. What is the case mix and CMI for these cases using the highest paying MS-DRGs?

Answers are in the Answer Key in the back of this book.

CPT Review

Review the beginning of each section in the CPT codebook for instructions about definitions and other information pertinent to assigning the correct code. The following are points to review:

Integumentary (Skin)

- Review the section on lacerations (repair) in the CPT book regarding when to add the lengths together and when to use an addition code for closure of the wound.
- Remember that grafts are measured in square centimeters, which is different than lacerations.
- Review the use of codes involved in excision, destruction, or other methods of removing lesions in the Malignant, Benign, Skin Tags, Other Lesions section.

Endoscopies

- In general, the Alphabetical Index will provide a range of codes for a given procedure. Some of these are open procedures. Make sure you look up each code before assigning it.
- There is a difference between "brushings and washings" and a biopsy in CPT.
    - Review the definitions of upper and lower gastrointestinal (GI) endoscopies in CPT
    - Upper gastrointestinal endoscopy
    - Proctosigmoidoscopy
    - Sigmoidoscopy
    - Colonoscopy
    - Review the Laparoscopy section of CPT
    - Review the definitions of the sinus procedures
    - Review the definitions under bronchoscopies. Remember that a bilateral bronchoscopy is coded twice or with a –50 modifier.

Musculoskeletal

- Review the terminology differences between ICD and CPT related to the treatment of fractures. For example, "manipulation" is the same in CPT as "reduction" in ICD-9.
- Understand the medical terminology, approaches, notes, and inclusions for knee repairs.

Outpatient Prospective Payment System

The outpatient prospective payment system (OPPS), for ambulatory care, began to be used for Medicare in August 2000. This system uses the ambulatory payment classifications (APCs) for reimbursement for hospital-based outpatient services such as outpatient surgery, emergency department visits, outpatient clinic visits, and outpatient ancillary tests. Some highlights of this system are listed here:

- APCs are similar to MS-DRGs in that they are both prospective payment methodologies and both have relative weights.
- APCs are different from MS-DRGs because outpatients can have multiple APCs for a given encounter, whereas an inpatient can have only one MS-DRG.
- APCs are generated for many services, such as x-rays, medical tests, clinic or emergency visits, surgical procedures, devices, drugs and biologicals, and partial hospitalizations.
- The billing number is the connecting identifier for a given patient's encounter that results in multiple APCs.

Status indicators denote what type of service was provided and assist in determining the payment. Status indicators include: X, ancillary; V, clinic or emergency department visit; T, significant procedure that is discounted when other T procedures are provided (the first procedure is paid at a rate of 100 percent whereas the second and those thereafter are paid at 50 percent); S, significant procedure that is paid at 100 percent and is not discounted; P, partial hospitalization; H, Pass-through device categories; G/J, drugs/biologicals; K, Non pass-through drugs and non-implantable biological, including therapeutic radiopharmaceuticals. Please visit the CMS web page (noted in the References in this book) for more information and a complete list of status indicators.

- CPT (numeric) and HCPCS (alphanumeric) modifiers approved for hospital outpatient are listed on the CPT codebook inside cover; –25, –27,–50, –52, –58, –59, –73, –74, –76, –77, –78, –79, –91, –LT, –RT, –CA, –E1, –E2, –E3, –E4, –FA, –F1, –F2, –F3, –F4, –F5, –F6, –F7, –F8, –F9, –GA, –GG, –GH, –LC, –LD, –QM, –QN, –RC, –TA, –T1, –T2, –T3, –T4, –T5, –T6, –T7, –T8, –T9.
- The following is a *hypothetical* example of one patient's APCs for a given encounter in the emergency department.

Billing Number	Status Indicator	CPT/HCPC	APC	Amount
789321	V	99284-25	0615	$223.17
789321	T	25500	0129	$111.73
789321	X	72050	0261	$75.23
789321	S	72128	0332	$195.07
789321	S	70450	0332	$195.07
			Reimbursement Total =	$800.27

While reviewing *Coding Clinic* and *CPT Assistant,* keep three goals in mind:

- Review the past three to five years of both references to prepare for the multiple choice and coding sections of the examination. Review at least the past three years of both references beginning with the most recent issue and reading backward (for instance, read 4th Quarter 2010, then 3rd Quarter 2010). This will allow you to know when changes occurred and what the most recent requirements are.
- Review as many topics that pertain to common inpatient and outpatient diagnoses and procedures for services that the average hospital would provide as you can. Be sure to read the fiscal year (FY) 2011 Official Coding Guidelines.
- Bolster knowledge in your areas of weakness that you have identified. The references used to develop the 2011 CCS exam stop at the end of 2010.

Ambulatory Payment Classifications (APCs)

It is important to understand the methodology of APCs. Some important issues to review are discounting, impact of CPT and HCPCS codes, medical necessity, the Correct Coding Initiative (CCI), status indicators, packaging, and the three-year transitional corridor. Refer to the Coding Challenges later in this section. AHIMA also has excellent resources regarding this topic. Also visit the CMS website for Medicare Program Memorandum.

Health Insurance Portability and Accountability Act (HIPAA)

Review recent AHIMA Practice Briefs and articles on this topic. Questions about HIPAA could be present on the exam. An easy way to study this area is to access information from the Body of Knowledge from the AHIMA CoP.

Common Diseases and Disorders with Associated Drugs

This is *not* a comprehensive list but can be helpful for review.

AIDS—Immunodeficiency syndrome caused by the human immunodeficiency virus (HIV). This disorder is associated with opportunistic infections, malignancies, and neurologic disease.
Medications: NRTIs-Nucleoside Reverse Transcriptase Inhibitors (Retrovir, AZT, Videx, ddl, Hivid, ddC, Zeril, d4tT, Epivir, 3TC); NRTIs-Nonnucleoside Reverse Transcriptase Inhibitors (Viramunde, Sustiva); Protease Inhibitors; (Invirase, Saquinavir, Crixovan, Indinavir, Kaletra, Lipinavir, Ritinavir)

Allergies—Hypersensitivity to a substance that does not normally cause a reaction.
Medications: antihistamines such as Claritin, Phenergan, Allegra, Zyrtec. The most common antihistamine for allergic reaction is diphenhydramine (Benadryl)

Anemia—Reduction in the number of circulating red blood cells or a reduction in the amount of hemoglobin in each red blood cell.
Medications: iron supplements, ferrous sulfate (Feosol), ferrous fumarate (Femiron), ferrous gluponate (Fergon); B_{12} (Cyanocobalamin); hematopoietic agents (Procrit, Epogen, Neupogen)

Angina pectoris—Severe pain associated with constriction in blood vessels to the heart with pain radiating to the left arm, abdomen, back, or jaw.
Medications: verapamil (Verelan, Calan SR); diltiazem (Cardizem CD, Dilacor); nifedipine (Adalat, Procardia); nitrates (Isordil, Imdur, ISMO); NTG-nitroglycerin (Nitroquick, Nitrodur); atenolom (Tenormin)

Anxiety—Mental disorder that manifests as fear, worry, or dread that is not related to a specific event or set of objects.
Medications: lorazepam (Ativan); alprazolam (Xanax); diazepam (Valium); paroxetine (Paxil); buspirone (Buspar)

Arrhythmia—Irregularities in the force or rhythm of the heart such as atrial fibrillation, tachycardia, bradycardia, or cardiac arrest.
Medications: verapamil (Calan SR, Verelan); digoxin (Lanoxin); quinidine (Quinaglute, Quinidex); amiodarone (Cordarone)

Arthritis—Inflammation of the joints. There are three major types of arthritis: osteoarthritis, rheumatoid arthritis, and gout.
Medications: ibuprofen (Advil, Motrin); hydrocortisone; Lodine; naproxen (Naprosyn; Oruvail; prednisone (Deltasone); Relafen; Voltaren; Medrol; Daypro; Celebrex

Asthma—Spasm of the bronchial tubes or swelling of the mucous membrane.
Medications: Albuterol (Proventil, Ventolin); theophylline; TheoDur; Serevent; Xopenea; Azmocort; Atroverit

Bipolar disorder—Mental disorder in which both mania and depression occur.
Medications: lithium; Lithobid; Eskalith; Zyprexa

Chronic obstructive pulmonary disease (COPD)—Group of disorders that decrease the ability of the lungs to provide ventilation to the body. Some forms of COPD include chronic obstructive asthma, chronic obstructive bronchitis, emphysema, bronchiectasis, and combinations of the aforementioned disorders.
Medications: Prednisone, albuterol (Proventil, Ventolin); Serevent; Alupent; Atrovent

Congestive heart failure (CHF)—Inability of the heart to pump the blood through the body adequately, resulting in edema in the extremities.
Medications: Bumex; Dyazide; furosemide (Lasix); HCTZ-hydrochlorothiazide; Lozol; digoxin (Lanoxin)

Dehydration—Loss of body fluid; this may be associated with severe nausea and vomiting, diarrhea, high fever, and urinary tract infections.
Medications: intravenous fluids, oral fluids; Pedialyte; Infalyte; Gatorade; Sportade

Depression—Mental disorder in which there is loss of interest in usually pleasurable pursuits.
Medications: amitriptyline hydrochloride (Elavil); Celexa; nortriptyline hydrochloride (Pamelor); Paxil; Prozac; trazodone hydrochloride (Desyrel); Zoloft

Diabetes mellitus—Disorder in which there is inadequate production or utilization of insulin. There are two types: Type I (the body does not produce or does not produce enough endogenous insulin) and Type II (the cells of the body do not utilize the endogenous insulin properly).
Medications: glyburide (DiaBeta, Glynase Prestab, Micronase); Glucophage, Glucotrol; insulin (Humulin, Humalog, Novolin), Lantus

Diverticulitis—Infection of the diverticula that causes inflammation.
Medications: antibiotics: ampicillin; gentamicin; tetracycline; cephalosporins (Mefoxin, Rocephin, Fortaz)

Diverticulosis—Formation of diverticula in the large intestine that can bleed or become infected or inflamed.
Medications: High-fiber diet

Fever—Elevated temperature.
Medications: acetaminophen (Tylenol); aspirin; ibuprofen (Motrin, Advil, Nuprin)

Gastrointestinal ulcers—Lesion in the mucosal membrane of the gastrointestinal tract that may cause bleeding or perforation. When a perforation occurs, the bacteria in the gastrointestinal tract may spill into the adjacent body cavity, causing peritonitis.
Medications: (Axid; Nexium; Pepcid; Prilosec; Tagamet; Zantac)

Hyperlipidemia—Excessive amount of lipids (fat) in the blood.
Medications: gemfibrozil (Lopid, Mevacor, Pravachol, Zocor, Lipitor)

Hypertension—Blood pressure that is persistently higher than normal. Malignant hypertension is characterized by severe vascular and other internal organ damage.
Medications: Altace; atenolol (Tenormin); Accupril; Capoten; Cardura; Coreg; Corgard; DynaCirc; enalapril (Vasotec); Hytrin; Lotensin; metropolol (Lopressor); Norvasc; Prinivil; Zestril

Hypokalemia—Potassium depletion in the blood.
Medications: potassium chloride (K-Dur, K-Lyte, Micro-K, Klor-Con, K-Tab, Kaon, K-Lor)

Hypotension—Persistently lower-than-normal blood pressure. There are two common forms of hypotension: orthostatic, and that due to other disorders such as anemia, trauma, hemorrhage, and fever.
Medications: volume expansion by increasing salt (NaCl); fludrocortisone acetate (Florinef Acetate); ephedrine

Hypothyroid—Decreased amount of thyroid secretion.
Medications: Levoxyl; Synthroid; thyroid; Levothroid; Cytomel

Impotence—Inability to maintain or achieve erection. This can occur because of an organic cause: following a radical prostatectomy, due to diabetes or alcohol abuse, or due to medications. Psychological reasons can also be a cause of this disorder.
Medications: Viagra; alprastadil (Muse, Edex, Caverject)

Infections—Result of an invasion of a pathogenic agent such as a virus or a bacterium. Infectious organisms include: bacteria (such as streptococci, staphylococci, spirochetes), viruses, fungi, and protozoa.
Medications: antibiotics; amoxicillin trihydrate (Amoxil); ampicillin; Augmentin; Bactroban;

Beepen-VK; Biaxin; Ceclor; Ceftin; Cefzil; cephalexin; Cipro; Claforan; Cotrim; doxycycline; Duricef; erythromycin (E.E.S., E-Mycin 333, Erythrcin, EryTab); Floxin; Fortaz; Lorabid; Macrobid; neomycin and polymixin; Penicillin VK; Pen-Vee K; Peridex; Principen; Rocephine; Suprax; tetracycline; Trimox; Vantin; Veetids; Zithromax; antifungals; Diflucan; Lotrisone; Nizoral; nystatin; antivirals; amvir; Valtrex; metronidazole; Zovirax

Malignant neoplasms—Uncontrolled growth of cells and the dispersion of malignant cells through the blood, the lymph system, or by direct extension to tissue adjacent to the tumor.
Medications: chemotherapy; 5-Fluorovracil; chlorambucil; cisplatin (Platinol); Cytoxan; doxorubicin (Adriamycin); Flutamide, megestrol acetate (Megace), MTX-methotrexate; prednisone; Taxol; Taxotere; vinblastine (Velban); vincristine (Oncovin); hormonal therapy; Arimidex; goserelin (Zoladex); Lupron; Proscar; Tamoxifen; biological response modifiers; Herceptin; Intron; Proleukin, IL-2; Roferon

Pneumonia or pneumonitis—Infection or inflammation of the lungs. There are multiple causes such as infectious agents (bacterial or virus), aspiration of secretions or food, inhalation of fumes, or radiation.
Medications: See Infections

Septicemia—Systemic infection usually manifesting in pathogenic organisms or accumulation of their toxins in the bloodstream.
Medications: See Infections

Thrombophlebitis—Inflammation of a vein. This condition leaves the patient at risk for embolisms.
Medication: warfarin sodium (Coumadin); heparin

Schizophrenia—Group of disorders characterized by disordered thinking, effect, and behavior.
Medications: haloperidol (Haldol); chlorpromazine (Thorazine); thioridazine (Mellaril); fluphenazine (Prolixin); Serentil; Seroquel; Clozaril; Zyprexa

Seizure—Involuntary muscular contractions and relaxations.
Medications: Depakote; Dilantin; Klonopin; Neurontin; phenobarbital; Tegretol; diazepam (Valium); Topamax

Coding Instructions (for the Exam)

Instructions and official guidelines for coding medical records are included in the following resources: ICD-9-CM, CPT, UHDDS, *Coding Clinic* for ICD-9-CM, and CPT Assistant. However, hospitals and other organizations may develop their own procedures in the absence of approved guidelines. To ensure consistent coding, the following procedures have been developed for use in the CCS exam. *These exam instructions do not supersede or replace official coding advice and guidelines included in the recommended exam study resources* (ahima.org/certification).

These instructions are to be used *only* in completing the CCS examination. They are provided to test takers as part of the exam booklet. Not adhering to these procedures may result in the miscoding of an exercise, which may result in the deduction of points when the item is scored.

Inpatient Coding

1. Apply UHDDS definitions, ICD-9-CM instructional notations and conventions, and current approved national ICD-9-CM coding guidelines to assign correct ICD-9-CM diagnostic and procedural codes to hospital inpatient medical records.
2. Sequence the ICD-9-CM codes, listing the principal diagnosis first.
3. Code other diagnoses that coexist at the time of admission, that develop subsequently, or that affect the treatment received and/or the length of stay. These represent additional conditions that affect patient care in terms of requiring clinical evaluation, therapeutic treatment, diagnostic procedures, extended length of hospital stay, or increased nursing care and/or monitoring (*ICD-9-CM Official Guidelines for Coding and Reporting* 2008).
   a. Code diagnoses that require active intervention during hospitalization. For example: Admission for small-bowel ileus and subsequent aspiration pneumonia that is treated with antibiotics and respiratory therapy. Code the ileus and aspiration pneumonia.
   b. Code diagnoses that require active management of chronic disease during hospitalization, which is defined as a patient who is continued on chronic management at time of hospitalization. For example: Admission for acute exacerbation of COPD. The patient has depression that extends the stay and for which psychiatric consultation is obtained. Code the COPD and depression. For example: Admission for acute exacerbation of COPD. Physician lists "history of depression" on face sheet, and the patient is given Desyrel. Code the COPD and depression.
   c. Code diagnoses of chronic systemic or generalized conditions that are not under active management when a physician documents them in the record and that may have a bearing on the management of the patient. For example: Admission for breast mass; diagnosis is carcinoma. Patient is blind and requires increased care. Code the breast carcinoma and blindness.
   d. Code status post previous surgeries or conditions likely to recur that may have a bearing on the management of the patient. For example: Admission for pneumonia; status post cardiac bypass surgery. Code the pneumonia and status post cardiac bypass surgery (V code).
   e. Do not code status post previous surgeries or histories of conditions that have no bearing on the management of the patient. For example: Admission for pneumonia; status post hernia repair six months prior to admission. Code only the pneumonia. *Previous surgeries involving transplants, internal devices, and prosthetics should be coded.*

f. Do not code localized conditions that have no bearing on the management of the patient. For example: Admission for hernia repair; the patient has a nevus on his leg that is not treated or evaluated. Code only the hernia and its repair.

g. Do not code abnormal findings (laboratory, x-ray, pathologic, and other diagnostic results) unless there is documentary evidence from the physician of their clinical significance. For example: Admission for elective joint replacement for degenerative joint disease. The laboratory report shows a serum sodium of 133; no further documentation addresses this laboratory result. Code only the degenerative joint disease and the replacement surgery. For example: Admission for elective joint replacement for degenerative joint disease. The laboratory report shows a low potassium level, and the physician documents hypokalemia. Intravenous potassium was administered by the physician for hypokalemia. Code the degenerative joint disease, the replacement surgery, and hypokalemia.

h. Do not code symptoms and signs that are characteristic of a diagnosis. For example: A patient has dyspnea due to COPD. Code only the COPD.

i. Do not code condition(s) in the Social History section that has no bearing on the management of the patient.

4. Do not assign External Cause of Injury and Poisoning Codes (E codes), except those that identify the causative substance for an adverse effect of a drug that is correctly prescribed and properly administered and/or poisoning (E850–E982).
5. Do not assign Morphology codes (M codes).
6. Code all procedures that fall within the code range 00.01–86.99, but do not code 57.94 (Foley catheter).
7. Do not code procedures that fall within the code range 87.01–99.99. But code procedures in the following ranges:

87.51–87.54	Cholangiograms
87.74 and 87.76	Retrogrades, urinary systems
88.40–88.58	Arteriography and angiography
92.21–92.29	Radiation therapy
94.24-94.27	Psychiatric therapy
94.61–94.69	Alcohol/drug detoxification and rehabilitation
96.04	Insertion of endotracheal tube
96.56	Other lavage of bronchus and trachea
96.70–96.72	Mechanical ventilation
98.51–98.59	ESWL
99.25	Chemotherapy

Ambulatory Care Coding

1. Apply ICD-9-CM instructional notations and conventions and current approved "Basic Coding Guidelines for Outpatient Services" and "Diagnostic Coding and Reporting Requirements for Physician Billing" (*Coding Clinic* 4th Quarter 1995, 1996) to select diagnoses, conditions, problems, or other reasons for care that require ICD-9-CM coding in an ambulatory care encounter/visit either in a hospital clinic, outpatient surgical area, emergency room, physician's office, or other ambulatory care setting.
2. Sequence the ICD-9-CM code so that the first diagnosis shown in the medical record is the one chiefly responsible for the outpatient services provided during the encounter/visit.
3. Code the secondary diagnoses as follows:
   a. Chronic diseases that are treated on an ongoing basis may be coded and reported as many times as the patient receives treatment and care for the condition(s).
   b. Code all documented conditions that coexist at the time of the encounter/visit that require or affect patient care, treatment, or management.
   c. Conditions previously treated and no longer existing should not be coded.
4. Do not assign External Cause of Injury and Poisoning Codes (E codes), except those that identify the causative substance for an adverse effect of a drug that is correctly prescribed and properly administered and/or poisoning (E850–E982).
5. Do not assign Morphology codes (M codes).
6. Do not assign ICD-9-CM procedure codes.
7. Assign CPT codes for all surgical procedures that fall in the surgery section.
8. Assign CPT codes from the following *only* if indicated on the case cover sheet:
   a. Anesthesia section
   b. Medicine section
   c. Evaluation and Management Services section
   d. Radiology section
   e. Laboratory and Pathology section
9. Assign CPT/HCPCS modifiers for hospital-based facilities, if applicable (regardless of payer).
10. Do not assign HCPCS Level II (alphanumeric) codes.

Evaluation and Management Mapping

The following map shows how a given facility has determined the criteria for evaluation and management (E/M) code assignment based on an emergency department record. Use the map to determine the correct codes for the emergency record that is provided. *Remember that each facility has the ability to develop its own mapping strategy. Therefore, the mapping scenario for the CCS exam will most likely be different from this one.* The purpose of this exercise is to practice using any mapping criteria that you are provided during the national exam. The following are the points need to determine the level of CPT code:

Level 1 = 1–20

Level 2 = 21–35

Level 3 = 36–47

Level 4 = 48–60

Level 5 = > 61

Critical Care > 61 with constant physician attendance

CPT Codes

Level 1 99281 99281–25 with procedure/laboratory/radiology

Level 2 99282 99282–25 with procedure/laboratory/radiology

Level 3 99283 99283–25 with procedure/laboratory/radiology

Level 4 99284 99284–25 with procedure/laboratory/radiology

Level 5 99285 99285–25 with procedure/laboratory/radiology

Emergency Department Acuity Points

	5	10	15	20	25
Meds Given	0-2	3-5	6-7	8-9	> 10
Extent of Hx	Brief	PF	EPF	Detail	Comprehensive
Extent of Exam	Brief	PF	EPF	Detail	Comprehensive
Number of Tests Ordered	0-1	2-3	4-5	6-7	> 8
Supplies Used	1	2-3	4-5	6-7	> 8

E/M MAPPING EXERCISE—EMERGENCY DEPARTMENT RECORD

DATE OF ADMISSION: 6/19 **DATE OF DISCHARGE:** 6/19

HISTORY (Problem Focused):

ADMISSION HISTORY: This 45-year-old African-American male was working in his office when he received news that his daughter, who is in the military, was deployed emergently to the Middle East. He began to have sharp pain in his right chest.

ALLERGIES: None

CHRONIC MEDICATIONS: None

FAMILY HISTORY: Noncontributory

SOCIAL HISTORY: The patient smokes one pack of cigarettes per day, but he does not smoke in the house.

REVIEW OF SYSTEMS: His integumentary, musculoskeletal, cardiovascular, genitourinary, and gastrointestinal systems are negative.

PHYSICAL EXAMINATION (Extended Problem Focused):

GENERAL APPEARANCE: This is an alert cooperative male in acute distress.

HEENT: PERRLA, extraocular movements are full

NECK: Supple

CHEST: Lungs are clear without rales or rhonchi. Heart has normal sinus rhythm.

ABDOMEN: Soft and nontender, no organomegaly

EXTREMITIES: Examination is normal

LABORATORY DATA: Urinalysis is normal, EKG normal, chest x-ray is normal. CBC and diff, cardiac enzymes show no abnormalities.

IMPRESSION: Noncardiac chest pain

TREATMENT: Patient was reassured, counseled to stop smoking, and referred to the clinic for smoking cessation and further management.

DISCHARGE DIAGNOSES: Noncardiac chest pain, possible anxiety reaction, smoking

DISCHARGE INSTRUCTIONS: The patient was instructed to make an appointment for the clinic tomorrow.

Answer the following questions:

1. What is the diagnostic code?
2. Based on the mapping scenario, what CPT code should be used?

(Answers can be found in the Answer Key in the back of this book.)

Coding Exercises

Code these cases in accordance with the exam coding instruction requirements listed earlier.

Inpatient

1. Admission for inguinal hernia repair. This 30-year-old patient has acquired immunodeficiency syndrome (AIDS) but is not symptomatic due to medication regimen. The procedure performed was a right indirect inguinal herniorrhaphy.
2. A 75-year-old male patient was admitted from a nursing home with dehydration and dysphagia due to a previous stroke. During hospitalization the patient was rehydrated and transferred back to the nursing home.
3. A patient is admitted to an acute care facility for detoxification from alcohol intoxication and barbiturate abuse with chronic alcoholism and barbiturate abuse. The patient also has cirrhosis of the liver due to alcoholism.
4. A 30-year-old patient was seen in the emergency department for repetitive epileptic seizures. The patient also had tic douloreux.
5. A patient was admitted to an acute care facility with a temperature of 102 and atrial fibrillation. The chest x-ray reveals pneumonia with subsequent documentation by the physician of pneumonia in the progress notes and discharge summary. The patient was treated with oral antiarrhythmia medications and IV antibiotics.
6. A patient with chronic cholecystitis and gallbladder stones underwent a laparoscopic cholecystectomy in an acute care facility. However, due to extensive gallbladder adhesions the procedure was converted to an open cholecystectomy.
7. A patient is admitted to the inpatient setting with hydronephrosis and a staghorn calculus of the kidney. The patient underwent an ureteroscopy with placement of ureteral stents and removal of calculus.
8. A 77-year-old nursing home patient was admitted to the acute care setting for excisional debridement of decubitus ulcer of the heel via surgical excision in the OR. The patient also has degenerative joint disease of both knees.
9. A 45-year-old woman was admitted to the inpatient setting for a displacement of a lumbar intervertebral disk. This was treated with a laminectomy and diskectomy.

10a. A 34-year-old woman delivered a live born, term baby boy with macrosomia. She had a hemorrhage following an episiotomy associated with low forceps prior to expulsion of the placenta.

10b. A single, newborn, term live-born baby boy.

11. Twin newborns, both born premature at 32 weeks via cesarean section, 1,002 g was the birth weight of the first twin whose mate was stillborn. The baby was admitted to the nursery from the delivery room. The baby also was treated for jaundice due to ABO incompatibility.
12. A patient is admitted to the acute care facility with chest pain. The patient was awakened from sleep; this was the patient's first experience with chest pain. The patient was given two nitroglycerin tablets in the emergency department. The chest pain was not relieved, resulting in the diagnosis of new onset unstable angina. Serial CPK was normal. Following a left cardiac catheterization and coronary angiography, the patient is found to have arteriosclerotic coronary artery disease.

13. This is the first admission for a patient with adenocarcinoma of the right lower lung who was also found with metastasis to the brain. The patient underwent a right lower lung lobectomy.
14. A patient has metastatic adenocarcinoma of bone.
15. A patient is admitted with metastatic carcinoma from breast to liver with previous mastectomy and no reoccurrence at the primary site.
16. A young woman was admitted after a car hit her from behind while she waited for a bus. She sustained a fractured fibula shaft and patella with a break in the skin at the mid-calf. The patient required an open reduction of the fibula fracture.
17. Syncope; bradycardia ruled out; due to taking Valium as prescribed by a physician. Patient also took an antihistamine as directed on the package without consulting a healthcare provider.
18. Sepsis due to the presence of an indwelling urinary catheter with a positive blood culture reflected in the progress notes of *Staphylococcus aureus* sepsis.
19. Respiratory distress syndrome, planned tracheotomy in 26-day-old baby.

Ambulatory/Outpatient

20. Noncardiac chest pain, esophageal acid reflux test.
21. Annual Screening mammogram.
22. Excision of basal cell carcinoma, 1.9-cm lesion left upper eyelid.
23. Hallux valgus repair with resection of the joint with implant in the first left toe proximal phalanx.
24. Metastatic ovarian cancer to the pleura. Thoracoscopic pleurodesis.
25. Symptomatic bradycardia due to sick sinus syndrome with replacement of dual chamber pacemaker generator with removal of old generator.
26. Esophagogastroduodenoscopy with sclerotherapy of esophageal varices.
27. Transurethral resection of the prostate for benign prostatic hypertrophy with electrocautery.
28. Cryosurgical destruction of simple papilloma of the penis.
29. Dysfunctional uterine bleeding for which hysteroscopy with endometrial ablation was undertaken.
30. Incompetent cervix with removal of cervical cerclage under spinal anesthesia in a pregnant woman.

CCS
Practice Questions

A blank answer sheet for these multiple choice questions can be found on page 45.

Domain 1: Health Information Documentation

1. An 84-year-old woman was admitted and discharged with hemiplegia and aphasia. A CT scan of the brain was performed which revealed an acute cerebral infarction and a possible small brain mass. After further testing, the patient was discharged with a final diagnosis of acute cerebral infarction. The condition(s) that should be coded are:

    a. Acute cerebral infarction

    b. Hemiplegia and aphasia

    c. Acute cerebral infarction, hemiplegia, and aphasia

    d. Possible brain mass, hemiplegia, and aphasia

2. A patient is discharged with a diagnosis of acute pulmonary edema due to congestive heart failure. What condition(s) should be coded?

    a. Acute pulmonary edema

    b. Congestive heart failure

    c. Acute pulmonary edema and congestive heart failure

    d. Unable to determine based on the information provided

3. The patient was admitted from the emergency department because of chest pain. Following blood work, it was determined that the CPK was elevated with MB enzymes elevated. The EKG shows nonspecific ST changes. What type of diagnosis might this be indicative of?

    a. Unstable angina

    b. Myocardial infarction

    c. Congestive heart failure

    d. Mitral valve stenosis

4. A patient is admitted and diagnosed with a fever and urinary burning. The discharge diagnosis is *Eschericia coli,* urosepsis. Which of the following represents the correct diagnoses and appropriate sequence of conditions?

    a. Fever, urinary burning, urosepsis

    b. Fever, urinary burning, sepsis

    c. *Eschericia coli,* urinary tract infection

    d. Urinary tract infection, *Eschericia coli*

5. A patient was admitted with heart failure within one week of a heart transplant. Due to the timing, the coder thought that it may represent a postoperative transplant rejection following heart transplant. What action (s) should the coding staff take?

   a. Query the physician.

   b. Assign the codes for the postoperative transplant rejection.

   c. Assign only the code for the transplant rejection.

   d. Assign only the code for heart failure.

6. A patient is admitted to a psychiatric unit of an acute-care facility. The patient experienced the following symptoms for most of the time almost every day for the last month: loss of interest or pleasure in most or all activities and this is a change from her prior level of functioning. She has also gained 15 lbs, has difficulty falling asleep, feels fatigued, and has difficulty making decisions. What potential diagnosis most closely fits the patient's overall symptoms?

   a. Insomnia

   b. Major depression

   c. Reye's syndrome

   d. Bipolar disorder

7. A patient is admitted to the hospital complaining of abdominal pain. Following evaluation, it was determined the patient had an intestinal obstruction due to adhesions from a prior abdominal surgery. The patient underwent an exploratory laparotomy with lysis of adhesions. What conditions should be coded?

   a. Abdominal pain, abdominal adhesions, abdominal obstruction, laparotomy, lysis of adhesions

   b. Abdominal adhesions, abdominal obstruction, postoperative complications of the digestive system, laparotomy, lysis of adhesions

   c. Abdominal adhesions with obstruction, lysis of adhesions

   d. Abdominal adhesions and abdominal obstruction, postoperative complications of the digestive system, lysis of adhesions

8. A patient's principal diagnosis is pneumonia (486) (MS-DRG 195). Which of the following may legitimately change the coding of the pneumonia in accordance with the UHDDS and relevant clinical documentation?

   a. Sputum culture reflects growth of normal flora.

   b. Patient has a positive gram stain.

   c. Patient is found to have dysphagia with aspiration.

   d. Patient has nonproductive sputum.

9. A patient is diagnosed with infertility due to endometriosis and undergoes a laparoscopic laser destruction of pelvic endometriosis. In order to code this encounter accurately, what steps must the coder take?
   a. Review the operative report to determine what procedure codes to use and also to determine the site or sites of endometriosis so codes with the highest specificity may be assigned, and use infertility as a principal diagnosis.
   b. Review the operative report to determine where the laser was used in the pelvis so the site or sites of endometriosis can be specified, and assign a principal diagnosis of infertility.
   c. Review the operative report to determine where the laser was used in the pelvis so the site or sites of endometriosis can be specified as principal, and assign a secondary diagnosis of infertility.
   d. Review the operative report to determine what procedure codes to use and also to determine the site or sites of endometriosis so codes with the highest specificity may be assigned, and use the diagnosis of infertility as a secondary condition.

Domain 2: Diagnosis Coding

10. A patient was given heparin during hospitalization for a deep vein thrombophlebitis of the right lower extremity. The patient had back pain and the nurse was not answering the bell, so he decided to take two aspirin. The interaction between the aspirin and heparin caused a subcutaneous hemorrhage of the thigh of the right lower extremity. How should the interaction between aspirin and heparin coded?
    a. Poisoning codes for aspirin and heparin, and subcutaneous hemorrhage of the thigh of the right lower extremity as secondary conditions
    b. Poisoning codes for aspirin and heparin, and subcutaneous hemorrhage of the thigh of the right lower extremity as principal
    c. Adverse effects of drugs for aspirin and heparin, and subcutaneous hemorrhage of the thigh of the right lower extremity as secondary conditions
    d. Adverse effects of drugs for aspirin and heparin as secondary diagnoses, and subcutaneous hemorrhage of the thigh of the right lower extremity as principal

11. A patient is admitted to the hospital for pain due to pacemaker electrode. The patient also has hypothyroidism due to partial thyroidectomy seven years ago and a breast cyst. The pacemaker electrode was relocated and synthroid was given during hospitalization. The diagnostic codes (excluding E codes) that should be assigned are:

996.0	Mechanical complication of cardiac device, implant, and graft
996.01	due to cardiac pacemaker (electrode)
996.6	Infection and inflammatory reaction due to internal prosthetic device, implant and graft
996.61	due to cardiac device, implant, and graft
996.7	Other complications of internal (biological) (synthetic) prosthetic device, implant, and graft
996.72	due to other cardiac device, implant, and graft
610.0	Solitary cyst of breast
610.4	Mammary duct ectasia
244.9	Unspecified hypothyroidism
244.0	Postsurgical hypothyroidism
244.1	Other postablative hypothyroidism
V45.79	Other acquired absence of organ

a. 996.01, 244.0
b. 996.61, 244.0, 610.0
c. 996.72, 244.0
d. 996.72, 244.0, 610.0

12. A patient was admitted to the emergency department for abdominal pain with diarrhea and was diagnosed with infectious gastroenteritis. The patient also had angina and chronic obstructive pulmonary disease. The diagnoses would be coded and sequenced as:

a. Abdominal pain, infectious gastroenteritis, chronic obstructive pulmonary disease, angina
b. Infectious gastroenteritis, chronic obstructive pulmonary disease, angina
c. Gastroenteritis, abdominal pain, angina
d. Diarrhea, chronic obstructive pulmonary disease, angina

13. A patient was admitted to the endoscopy unit for a screening colonoscopy. During the colonoscopy, polyps of the colon were found and a polypectomy was performed. What diagnostic codes should be used and how should they be sequenced?

V76	Special screening for malignant neoplasms
V76.51	Colon
211	Benign neoplasm of other parts of digestive system
211.3	Benign neoplasm of colon

a. V76.51

b. 211.3

c. V76.51, 211.3

d. 211.3, V76.51

Please refer to the following when answering questions 14 and 15.

216 Benign neoplasm of skin

Includes: Blue nevus
dermatofibroma
hydrocystoma
pigmented nevus
syringoadenoma
syringoma

Excludes:
Skin of genital organs (221.0–222.9)

14. When coding benign neoplasm of the skin, the section noted above directs the coder to:

a. Use category 216 for a syringoma.

b. Use category 216 for malignant melanoma.

c. Use category 216 for malignant neoplasm of the bone.

d. Use category 216 for malignant neoplasm of the skin.

15. When coding benign neoplasm of the skin of the labia, the section noted above directs the coder to:

a. Use category 216

b. Use category 221.0–222.9

c. Use category 174

d. Use category 173

16. A patient was discharged from the same-day-surgery unit with the following diagnoses: mature senile cataract, diabetes mellitus, hypertension, and was treated for mild acute renal failure. Which codes are correct?

250.00	Diabetes mellitus without mention of complication
250.40	Diabetes with renal manifestations
366.1	Senile cataract
366.10	Senile cataract, unspecified
366.17	Total or mature cataract
401.9	Essential Hypertension, unspecified
403.90	Hypertensive chronic kidney disease, unspecified
584.9	Acute kidney failure, unspecified

a. 366.10, 250.40, 403.90, 584.9

b. 366.17, 250.00, 401.9, 584.9

c. 366.17, 250.40, 403.90, 584.9

d. 366.10, 250.00, 401.9, 584.9

17. A patient is admitted with an acute exacerbation of COPD with stage V hypertensive kidney disease. What is the correct diagnostic code assignment?

403.90	Hypertensive chronic kidney disease unspecified with chronic kidney disease stage I through stage IV or unspecified
403.91	Hypertensive chronic kidney disease unspecified with chronic kidney disease stage V or end-stage renal disease
491.21	Obstructive chronic bronchitis with (acute) exacerbation
496	Chronic airway obstruction, not elsewhere classified
585.5	Chronic kidney disease, stage V

a. 496, 403.90

b. 491.21, 403.90

c. 496, 403.91

d. 491.21, 403.91, 585.5

18. A patient is admitted with acute respiratory failure, hypertension, and congestive heart failure. The patient was intubated upon admission to the hospital.

401.9	Essential hypertension, unspecified
428.0	Congestive heart failure, unspecified
518.81	Acute respiratory failure
518.82	Other pulmonary insufficiency, NEC
518.83	Chronic respiratory failure
518.84	Acute and chronic respiratory failure
518.89	Other disease of lung, NEC

a. 518.81, 401.9, 428.0

b. 428.0, 518.81, 401.9

c. 518.84, 401.9, 428.0

d. 428.0, 518.84, 401.9

19. A patient is treated for esophageal varices with hemorrhage due to cirrhosis. The diagnostic codes that would be assigned are:

456.0	Esophageal varices with bleeding
456.1	Esophageal varices without mention of bleeding
456.20	Esophageal varices in diseases classified elsewhere with bleeding
456.21	Esophageal varices in diseases classified elsewhere without mention of bleeding
571.5	Cirrhosis of the liver without mention of alcohol

a. 456.0, 571.5

b. 456.20, 571.5

c. 571.5, 456.0

d. 571.5, 456.20

20. Normal pregnancy and delivery with loose nuchal cord around neck. Delivery was accompanied by an episiotomy with birth of liveborn male infant. Delivery room record states "no evidence of fetal problem." What diagnostic and procedure codes should be assigned?

650	Normal delivery
663.11	Cord around neck, with compression, delivered with or without mention of antepartum condition
663.12	Cord around neck, with compression, delivered with mention of postpartum condition
663.31	Other and unspecified cord entanglement, without mention of compression, delivered with or without mention of antepartum condition
663.32	Other and unspecified cord entanglement, without mention of compression, delivered with mention of postpartum condition
V27.0	Single liveborn
73.59	Other manually assisted delivery
73.6	Episiotomy

a. 650, V27.0, 73.6
b. 663.31, V27.0, 73.6
c. 663.31, 73.6
d. 663.31, V27.0, 73.59

21. Normal twin delivery at 30 weeks. Both babies were delivered vaginally and were liveborn. What conditions should have codes assigned?

644.21	Early onset of delivery, delivered with or without mention of antepartum condition
650	Normal delivery
651.01	Twin pregnancy, delivered with or without mention of antepartum condition
V27.0	Single liveborn
V27.2	Twins, both liveborn

a. 650, V27.0
b. 644.21, V27.2
c. 651.01, 644.21, V27.2
d. 650, 651.01, V27.2

Domain 3: Procedure Coding

22. A patient was treated in the emergency department with lacerations of the neck and underwent a repair of two (2) wounds of the neck (2.0 cm and 1.4 cm) with layered closure. What are the diagnostic (excluding E codes) and procedure codes assigned?

874.8	Open wound of neck, Other and unspecified parts, without mention of complication
874.9	Open wound of neck, Other and unspecified parts, with complicated
86.59	Closure of skin and subcutaneous tissue of other sites
12041	Repair, intermediate, wounds of neck, hands, feet and/or external genitalia; 2. 5 cm or less
12042	Repair, intermediate, wounds of neck, hands, feet, and/or external genitalia, 2.6 cm to 7.5 cm

a. 874.8, 86.59

b. 874.9, 86.59

c. 874.8, 12041

d. 874.8, 12042

23. A 12-year boy was seen in an ambulatory surgical center for pain in his right arm. The x-ray showed fracture of ulna. Patient underwent closed reduction of fracture right proximal ulna. What diagnostic and procedure codes should be assigned?

813	Fracture of radius and ulna
813.04	Other and unspecified fractures of proximal end of ulna (alone)
79.02	Closed reduction of fracture without internal fixation; radius and ulna
25560	Closed treatment of radial and ulnar shaft fracture, without manipulation
24670	Closed treatment of ulnar fracture, proximal end (eg, olecranon or coronoid process(es)); without manipulation
24675	Closed treatment of ulnar fracture, proximal end (eg, olecranon or coronoid process(es)); with manipulation

a. 813, 79.02

b. 813.04, 79.02

c. 813.04, 25560

d. 813.04, 24675

24. Assign the code(s) for Endoscopic sinusotomy with bilateral anterior ethmoidectomy.

31231	Nasal endoscopy, diagnostic, unilateral or bilateral
31254	Nasal/sinus endoscopy, surgical; with ethmoidectomy, partial (anterior)
-50	Bilateral procedure

a. 31254

b. 31254–50

c. 31254, 31254

d. 31231

25. Assign the code(s) for Bronchoscopy with bilateral transbronchial biopsy.

31628	Bronchoscopy, rigid or flexible, including fluoroscopic guidance, when performed; with transbronchial lung biopsy(s), single lobe
31629	Bronchoscopy, rigid or flexible, including fluoroscopic guidance, when performed; with transbronchial needle aspiration biopsy(s), trachea, main stem and/or lobar bronchus(i)
31632	Bronchoscopy, rigid or flexible, including fluoroscopic guidance, when performed; with transbronchial lung biopsy(s), each additional lobe
-50	Bilateral procedure

a. 31628

b. 31628–50

c. 31628, 31632

d. 31629

26. Assign the code(s) for Diagnostic left and right cardiac catheterization, left ventriculogram, coronary arteriogram.

37.21	Right heart cardiac catheterization
37.22	Left heart cardiac catheterization
37.23	Combined right and left heart cardiac catheterization
88.53	Angiocardiography of left heart structures
88.54	Combined right and left heart angiocardiography
88.55	Coronary arteriography using a single catheter
88.56	Coronary arteriography using two catheters
88.57	Other and unspecified coronary arteriography

a. 37.21, 37.22, 88.53, 88.55

b. 37.23, 88.57, 88.53

c. 37.23

d. 88.53, 88.55, 37.23

27. Assign the code for Dilatation and curettage for missed abortion at 11 weeks' gestation.

69.01	Dilation and curettage for termination of pregnancy
69.02	Dilation and curettage following delivery or abortion
69.09	Other dilation and curettage
69.51	Aspiration curettage of uterus for termination of pregnancy

a. 69.02

b. 69.01

c. 69.09

d. 69.51

28. Bilateral epidural lumbar injection of steroids:

62282	Injection/infusion of neurolytic substance (eg, alcohol, phenol, iced saline solutions) with or without other therapeutic substance; epidural, lumbar, sacral (caudal)
62311	Injection, single (not via indwelling catheter), not including neurolytic substances, with or without contrast, (for either localization or epidurography), of diagnostic or therapeutic substance(s) (including anesthetic, antispasmodic, opioid, steroid, other solution), epidural or subarachnoid; lumbar, sacral (caudal)
-50	Bilateral procedure

a. 62282

b. 62311

c. 62311, 62311

d. 62311–50

29. Assign the code(s) for Extraction of extracapsular cataract with simultaneous intraocular lens insertion in the right eye.

66982	Extracapsular cataract removal with insertion of intraocular lens prosthesis (1-stage procedure), manual or mechanical technique (eg, irrigation and aspiration or phacoemulsification), complex requiring devices or techniques not generally used in routine cataract surgery (eg, iris expansion device, suture support for intraocular lens, or primary posterior capsulorrhexis), or performed on patients in the amblyogenic developmental stage
66983	Intracapsular cataract extraction with insertion of intraocular lens prosthesis (1-stage procedure)
66984	Extracapsular cataract removal with insertion of intraocular lens prosthesis (1-stage procedure), manual or mechanical technique (eg, irrigation and aspiration or phacoemulsification)
-51	Multiple procedures
-RT	Right side

a. 66982–RT

b. 66983–RT

c. 66984–RT

d. 66984–51

30. Assign the code(s) for Chemotherapy for 3 hours' infusion.

96401	Chemotherapy administration, subcutaneous or intramuscular; non-hormonal anti-neoplastic
96413	Chemotherapy administration, intravenous infusion technique; up to 1 hour, single or initial substance/drug
+96415	each additional hour (List separately in addition to code for primary procedure.)
-51	Multiple procedures

a. 96413, 96415, 96415

b. 96413, 96415–51

c. 96413, 96413, 96413

d. 96401

31. Assign the code(s) for Chest x-ray, complete.

71010	Radiologic examination, chest; single view, frontal
71020	Radiologic examination, chest, 2 views, frontal and lateral
71030	Radiologic examination, chest, complete, minimum 4 views
71035	Radiologic examination, chest, special views (eg, lateral decubitus, Bucky studies)

a. 71020

b. 71030

c. 71010, 71035

d. 71035

32. Assign the code(s) for Mammographic guidance for breast needle localization placement with fine needle aspiration.

77031	Stereotactic localization guidance for breast biopsy or needle placement (eg, for wire localization or for injection), each lesion, radiological supervision and interpretation
77032	Mammographic guidance for needle placement, breast (eg, for wire localization or for injection), each lesion, radiological supervision and interpretation
10021	Fine needle aspiration, without imaging guidance
10022	Fine needle aspiration, with imaging guidance

a. 77032

b. 10022

c. 77032, 10022

d. 77031

33. A laparoscopic tubal ligation is completed. What is the correct CPT code assignment?

49320	Laparoscopy, abdomen, peritoneum, and omentum, diagnostic, with or without collection of specimen(s) by brushing or washing
58662	Laparoscopy, surgical; with fulguration or excision of lesions of the ovary, pelvic viscera, or peritoneal surface by any method
58670	Laparoscopy, surgical; with fulguration of oviducts (with or without transection)
58671	Laparoscopy, surgical; with occlusion of oviducts by device (eg, band, clip, or Falope ring)

a. 49320, 58662

b. 58670

c. 58671

d. 49320

Domain 4: Regulatory Guidelines and Reporting Requirements for Acute-Care (Inpatient) Service

34. Hospital A: The patient is admitted for chest pain and is found to have an acute inferior myocardial infarction with atrial fibrillation. After the atrial fibrillation was controlled and the patient was stabilized, the patient was transferred to Hospital B for a CABG X3. The appropriate sequencing and ICD codes for both hospitalizations would be:

410.41	Acute myocardial infarction of other inferior wall, initial episode of care
410.42	Acute myocardial infarction of other inferior wall, subsequent episode of care
410.91	Acute myocardial infarction of unspecified site, initial episode of care
410.92	Acute myocardial infarction of unspecified site, subsequent episode of care
427.31	Atrial fibrillation
786.50	Chest pain, unspecified
36.13	Aortocoronary bypass of three coronary arteries

a. Hospital A: 786.50, 410.91, 427.31: Hospital B: 410.92, 427.31, 36.13

b. Hospital A: 410.41, 427.31: Hospital B: 410.92, 427.31, 36.13

c. Hospital A: 410.41, 427.31: Hospital B: 410.41, 427.31, 36.13

d. Hospital A: 410.42, 427.31: Hospital B: 410.41, 427.31, 36.13

35. A patient is admitted and discharged with chest pain. After evaluation, it is suspected the patient may have gastroesophageal reflux disease (GERD). The final diagnosis was "Rule out GERD." The correct code assignment would be:

a. V71.7, Observation for suspected cardiovascular disease

b. 789.01, Abdominal pain, right upper quadrant

c. 530.81, Esophageal reflux

d. 786.50, Chest pain, unspecified

36. If a patient has a principal diagnosis of septicemia, which of the following procedures will increase the DRG assignment the most?

a. Bronchoscopy with biopsy (33.24)

b. Debridement of nails (86.27)

c. Nonexcisional debridement of skin ulcer with abrasion (86.28)

d. Ventilator management for 106 consecutive hours (96.72)

37. A patient presents to a facility with a history of prostate cancer and mental confusion on admission. The patient completed radiation therapy for prostatic carcinoma three years ago and is status post a radical resection of the prostate. A CT scan of the brain reveals metastatic carcinoma of the brain. The correct coding and sequencing of this patient's record is:

 a. Metastatic carcinoma of the brain, carcinoma of the prostate, mental confusion
 b. Mental confusion, history of carcinoma of the prostate, admission for chemotherapy
 c. Metastatic carcinoma of the brain, history of carcinoma of the prostate
 d. Carcinoma of the prostate, metastatic carcinoma to the brain

38. The patient is discharged with hemiplegia and aphasia associated with a cerebral infarction of the left side of the brain. The patient is right handed and also has compensated congestive heart failure and a history of hypertension (both conditions currently controlled on medication and treated while in the hospital). What code assignment would be appropriate?

342.90	Hemiplegia, unspecified, affecting unspecified side
342.91	Hemiplegia, unspecified, affecting dominant side
342.92	Hemiplegia, unspecified affecting nondominant side
434.90	Cerebral artery occlusion unspecified, without mention of cerebral infarction
434.91	Cerebral artery occlusion unspecified, with cerebral infarction
401.9	Essential hypertension, unspecified
428.0	Congestive heart failure, unspecified
784.3	Aphasia

 a. 434.91, 342.91, 784.3, 428.0, 401.9
 b. 342.90, 784.3, 428.0, 401.9
 c. 434.90, 342.90, 784.3
 d. 434.91, 342.90, 784.3

39. A patient is admitted with a chronic productive cough with hemoptysis. A bronchoscopy with transbronchial biopsy of the lower lobe was undertaken that revealed squamous cell carcinoma. Which conditions should be identified as present on admission?

786.2	Cough
786.3	Hemoptysis
162.5	Malignant neoplasm of lower lobe, bronchus or lung

 a. 162.5
 b. 786.2, 786.3
 c. 162.5, 786.3
 d. 162.5, 786.2, 786.3

Domain 5: Regulatory Guidelines and Reporting Requirements for Outpatient Services

40. Carcinoma of multiple overlapping sites of the bladder. Diagnostic cystoscopy and transurethral fulguration of bladder lesions (1.9 cm, 6.0 cm) are completed and a skin lesion was also removed from the left thigh. What modifier should be added to the procedure codes?

    a. –50, Bilateral procedure

    b. –51, Multiple procedures

    c. –59, Distinct procedure service

    d. –99, Multiple modifiers

41. A bronchoscopy with biopsy of the left bronchus was completed and revealed adenocarcinoma. What modifier should be added to the procedure codes?

    a. –22, Increased procedural services

    b. –51, Multiple procedures

    c. –59, Distinct procedure service

    d. No modifiers should be reported.

42. Wide excision of 0.65-cm malignant melanoma (margins included) from right forearm. The diagnosis and procedure codes reported are:

172.6	Malignant melanoma of skin; upper limb, including shoulder
195.4	Malignant neoplasm of upper limb
11401	Excision, benign lesion including margins, except skin tag (unless listed elsewhere), trunk, arms, or legs; excised diameter 0.6 to 1.0 cm
11601	Excision, malignant lesion including margins, trunk, arms, or legs; excised diameter 0.6 to 1.0 cm
25075	Excision, tumor, soft tissue of forearm and/or wrist area; subcutaneous, less than 3 cm

    a. 172.6, 11401

    b. 195.4, 11601

    c. 172.6, 11601

    d. 172.6, 25705

43. Colonoscopy with cauterization of diverticular bleeding. What diagnoses and procedures should be reported?

578.9	Hemorrhage of gastrointestinal tract, unspecified
562.10	Diverticulosis of colon (without mention of hemorrhage)
562.12	Diverticulosis of colon with hemorrhage
563.13	Diverticulitis of colon with hemorrhage
45378	Colonoscopy, flexible, proximal to splenic flexure, diagnostic, with or without collection of specimen(s) by brushing or washing, with or without colon decompression (separate procedure)
45382	Colonoscopy, flexible, proximal to splenic flexure; with control of bleeding (eg, injection, bipolar cautery, unipolar cautery, laser, heater probe, stapler, plasma, coagulator)

a. 562.10, 578.9, 45382

b. 562.12, 45382

c. 563.13, 45382

d. 578.9, 562.10, 45382

44. Recurrent left inguinal hernia with laparoscopic repair. What diagnoses and procedures should be reported?

550.91	Inguinal hernia, without mention of obstruction or gangrene, unilateral or unspecified, recurrent
550.10	Inguinal hernia, with obstruction, without mention of gangrene, unilateral or unspecified (not specified as recurrent)
550.11	Inguinal hernia, with obstruction, without mention of gangrene, unilateral or unspecified, recurrent
49520	Repair recurrent inguinal hernia, any age, reducible
49521	Repair recurrent inguinal hernia, any age, reducible, incarcerated or stangulated
49651	Laparoscopy, surgical, repair recurrent inguinal hernia

a. 550.91, 49520

b. 550.11, 49521

c. 550.91, 49651

d. 550.10, 49520

45. A patient was admitted after a fall down a series of steps. The patient was unconscious for approximately 45 minutes and was admitted to the emergency department (ED) within 3 hours of the fall. A CT scan was performed within an hour of admission to the ED. A skull vault fracture with cerebral contusion was diagnosed by the ED physician based on the findings in the CT scan. What conditions should be reported on the Unified Billing form 04 (UB-04)?

780.09	Alterations of consciousness; other (drowsiness, semicoma, unconsciousness, somnolence, stupor)
800.12	Fracture of vault of skull, closed with cerebral laceration and contusion, with brief (less than 1 hour) loss of consciousness
803.12	Other and unqualified skull fractures, closed with cerebral laceration and contusion, with brief (less than 1 hour) loss of consciousness
803.42	Other and unqualified skull fractures, closed with intracranial injury of other and unspecified nature, with brief (less than 1 hour) loss of consciousness
851.82	Other and unspecified cerebral laceration and contusion, without mentioning of open intracranial wound, with brief (less than 1 hour) loss of consciousness
V71.4	Observation following other accident
E880.9	Fall on or from stairs or steps; other stairs or steps
E849.9	Place of occurrence, unspecified place
87.03	Computerized axial tomography of head

a. 800.12, E880.9

b. 780.09, 87.03

c. 803.02, 87.03, E880.9, E849.9

d. 800.12, E880.9, E849.9, 87.03

Domain 6: Data Quality and Management

46. A 64-year-old female was discharged with the final diagnosis of acute renal failure and hypertension. What coding rule applies?

a. Use combination code of hypertension and renal failure.

b. Use separate codes for hypertension and chronic renal failure.

c. Use separate codes for hypertension and acute renal failure.

d. Use separate codes for elevated blood pressure and chronic renal failure.

47. Cystourethroscopy with removal of two lesions of separate locations in the bladder, one is 1.5-cm bladder tumor anterior wall and one is 0.75-cm in the lateral wall. What coding rule applies?
    a. Two CPT codes should be used with a modifier –59.
    b. Two CPT codes should be used.
    c. Code only the CPT code for cystourethroscopy.
    d. Code only the largest tumor.

48. Diagnostic-related groups (DRGs) and ambulatory patient classifications (APCs) are similar in that they are both:
    a. Determined by HCPCS codes
    b. Focused on hospital outpatients
    c. Focused on hospital inpatients
    d. Prospective payment systems

Please refer to the following data when answering questions 49 and 50 (*Note:* The DRG numbers and weights are not actual numbers and weights for fiscal year 2011.)

MS-DRG	MS-DRG Wt.	Number of Patients
191	2.0	10
192	1.5	10
193	1.0	10

49. The case-mix index for the information provided above is:
    a. 0.679
    b. 0.89
    c. 1.5
    d. 0.75

50. The information provided shows that:
    a. The payment is higher for patients with DRG 191.
    b. There are more patients with DRG 191.
    c. The case-mix index could be increased if more patients in DRG 193 were admitted.
    d. The case mix would not increase if more patients in DRG 193 were admitted.

Domain 7: Information and Communication Technologies

51. A surgeon would like to undertake a research study on his patients with stage II malignant melanoma of the back, who have undergone wide excision of the melanoma. What work processes and associated software could be used to provide this information?

    a. Obtain a summary of the cases from the cancer registry, import them into a spreadsheet, and provide to the surgeon.

    b. Obtain a summary of the cases from the chart completion software, import them into a spreadsheet, and provide to the surgeon.

    c. Obtain a summary of the cases from the master patient index, import them into a spreadsheet, and provide to the surgeon.

    d. Obtain a summary of the cases from the transcription tracking software, import them into a spreadsheet, and provide to the surgeon.

52. The coding supervisor is concerned that patients diagnosed with carcinoid colon tumors were miscoded as malignant during the last six months. To address this situation, what work processes could be undertaken?

    a. Obtain the cases of carcinoid colon tumors from the cancer registry, obtain the cases of malignant colon tumors from the billing system, import both lists into a spreadsheet, and compare them. The cases in the cancer registry and not in the billing system are likely malignant and should be manually reviewed.

    b. Compare the cases from the chart completion software with the billing software. Identify the cases that are not in the billing system. These cases should be manually reviewed to ensure they are not carcinoid tumors.

    c. Obtain the cases of malignant colon tumors from both the cancer registry and the billing system; import both lists into a spreadsheet and compare them. Identify the cases that are not in the tumor registry that are in the billing system. These cases should be manually reviewed to ensure they are not carcinoid tumors.

    d. Compare the cases from the transcription tracking software to the billing system. Identify the cases that are not in the transcription tracking software and are in the billing system. These cases should be manually reviewed to ensure they are not carcinoid tumors.

53. A quality improvement study showed that newborn codes associated with maternal conditions are not being coded as often as they should. What HIM software could be used to identify the mother's chart so it can be reviewed at the time the newborn record is coded?

    a. Birth certificate registry or master patient index

    b. Transcription registry or correspondence registry

    c. Quality improvement or operative registry

    d. Pathology or laboratory information

Domain 8: Privacy, Confidentiality, Legal, and Ethical Issues

54. A facility located near a national park has a significant number of snake bites and patients receive treatment with antivenom in urgent-care settings. Sometimes a patient is admitted to the hospital after several days. Can the urgent-care setting provide the hospital with a list of names of patients treated with snake antivenom?
    a. Only the names of patients who are admitted to the hospital can be requested if the physician needs it for continuity of care, but an entire list of patients cannot be provided.
    b. A list of names could be provided.
    c. No information can be obtained under any circumstances.
    d. A list of patients may be available after consultation with the national park ranger.

55. When patients are admitted with vaginal bleeding, one of the financial analysts has determined that if one additional procedure code were routinely added to each case, reimbursement would be increased. This would be considered an ethical practice if:
    a. The vice president of finance approves the procedure.
    b. The billing department wants this, it can be done.
    c. Under no circumstances could this be done.
    d. There is documentation of the procedure in the medical record.

56. The patient was admitted for breast carcinoma in the right breast at two o'clock. This was removed via lumpectomy. The patient was found to have 1 of 7 lymph nodes positive for carcinoma during axillary lymph node dissection. One of the patient's neighbors who is also a coworker at the hospital called the coding department to get the patient's diagnosis because she is a cancer survivor herself. The coder should:
    a. Discuss the case with the coworker.
    b. Report the incident to hospital security.
    c. Give the caller false information.
    d. Explain that discussing the case would violate the patient's right to privacy.

57. The billing department has requested that copies of the final coding summary with codes and associated code meanings for Medicare be printed remotely in the admission department. Currently they request the summaries only when there is an unspecified procedure. Each time the coding supervisor goes to the admission department, the coding summaries have been left on a table near the patient entrance. Of the actions presented here, what action is the best one the coding supervisor should take?
    a. Comply with the request.
    b. Refuse to undertake this without further explanation.
    c. Ignore the request.
    d. Explain to the billing department supervisor that leaving the coding summary in public view violates the patient's right to privacy.

Domain 9: Compliance

58. Inpatients who undergo open reduction and internal fixation of the femur because of a fracture are routinely coded with blood loss anemia because of a policy that specifies that this should be done when there is intraoperative blood loss of 500 CCs or more documented in the operative report and the patient has a low hemoglobin. Why is this correct or incorrect?

    a. It is correct to code blood loss anemia because the policy requires it.

    b. It is correct because the clinical signs are documented in the record.

    c. It is incorrect because the patient must also have a blood transfusion in order for blood loss anemia to be coded.

    d. It is incorrect because the physician did not document the blood loss anemia in the progress notes.

59. A female patient is admitted for a second-degree cystocele. A repair is performed. In order to code this accurately, what document provides the required additional information?

    a. History and physical

    b. Discharge summary

    c. Consultation

    d. Operative report

60. In order to accurately code a cardiac catheterization, what needs to be determined based on review of documentation?

    a. The approach and the side of the heart (chambers) into which the catheter was inserted

    b. The approach, the side of the heart (chambers) into which the catheter was inserted, as well as any additional procedures performed

    c. The duration of the procedure

    d. If there is documentation of the procedure in the medical record that stents are considered

Multiple Choice Practice Answers

1. ______________
2. ______________
3. ______________
4. ______________
5. ______________
6. ______________
7. ______________
8. ______________
9. ______________
10. ______________
11. ______________
12. ______________
13. ______________
14. ______________
15. ______________
16. ______________
17. ______________
18. ______________
19. ______________
20. ______________
21. ______________
22. ______________
23. ______________
24. ______________
25. ______________
26. ______________
27. ______________
28. ______________
29. ______________
30. ______________
31. ______________
32. ______________
33. ______________
34. ______________
35. ______________
36. ______________
37. ______________
38. ______________
39. ______________
40. ______________
41. ______________
42. ______________
43. ______________
44. ______________
45. ______________
46. ______________
47. ______________
48. ______________
49. ______________
50. ______________
51. ______________
52. ______________
53. ______________
54. ______________
55. ______________
56. ______________
57. ______________
58. ______________
59. ______________
60. ______________

CCS
Practice Case Studies

Note: Review the Coding Instructions (for the Exam) in the Introduction of this book.

AMBULATORY CASE—PATIENT 1
FACE SHEET

DATE OF ADMISSION: 4/5 **DATE OF DISCHARGE:** 4/5

SEX: Male **AGE:** 37 **DISCHARGE DISPOSITION:** Home

ADMISSION DIAGNOSIS: Left inguinal hernia

DISCHARGE DIAGNOSIS: Same

PROCEDURES: Left inguinal herniorrhaphy with excision of lipoma of spermatic cord

HISTORY AND PHYSICAL EXAMINATION—PATIENT 1

ADMITTED: 4/5
HISTORY OF PRESENT ILLNESS: The patient has been well until several months ago when he began to have pain when lifting.
PAST MEDICAL HISTORY: The patient has no other significant medical or surgical history.
SOCIAL HISTORY: The patient does not use alcohol or tobacco.
ALLERGIES: No known allergies
MEDICATIONS: None
REVIEW OF SYSTEMS:
SKIN: Warm and dry, mucous membranes moist
HEENT: Essentially normal
LUNGS: Clear to percussion and auscultation
HEART: Normal, regular rhythm
ABDOMEN: Normal
GENITALIA: Palpable mass in inguinal canal
RECTAL: Normal
EXTREMITIES: No edema
NEUROLOGIC: Deep tendon reflexes normal
IMPRESSION: Left inguinal hernia
PLAN: Surgical repair of inguinal hernia

PROGRESS NOTES—PATIENT 1

DATE	NOTE
4/5	Nursing: Betadine scrub performed, patient anxious to get surgery over; preoperative medications given as ordered.
4/5	Attending MD: Brief op note Dx: Left inguinal hernia Px: Left inguinal herniorrhaphy Anes: Local plus sedation Complications: None
4/5	Attending MD: No bleeding; patient okay for discharge.

OPERATIVE REPORT—PATIENT 1

DATE: 4/5

PREOPERATIVE DIAGNOSIS: Left direct inguinal hernia

POSTOPERATIVE DIAGNOSIS: Left direct inguinal hernia

OPERATION: Left inguinal herniorrhaphy

ANESTHESIA: Local plus sedation

OPERATIVE INDICATIONS: A wide mouth direct sac was present in the lower inguinal canal. A lipoma of the cord was present, but no indirect sac.

OPERATIVE PROCEDURE: Under local anesthesia consisting of the equivalent of 19 cc of 1% Xylocaine and 8 cc of 0.5% Marcaine, the abdomen was prepared with Betadine and sterilely draped. A left inguinal incision was made and carried down through subcutaneous tissues to the aponeurosis of the external oblique, which was opened from the external ring to a point over the internal ring. Flaps were cleaned in both directions. The nerve was retracted inferiorly. The cord structures were separated from the surrounding at the level of the pubic tubercle and retracted with a Penrose drain. Cremaster over the cord was opened and a search made for an indirect sac. None was found. Lipoma of the cord was dissected free and clamped at its base and excised. The base was ligated with 00 chromic catgut. Additional cremasteric muscles were divided and ligated with 00 chromic catgut. The direct sac was further dissected down to its base and inverted as the defect was closed by approximating transversus to transversus with a running suture of 00 Vicryl. The floor of the canal was then closed by approximating the internal oblique to the shelving portion of the inguinal ligament with multiple sutures of 0 Ethibond. The external oblique aponeurosis was then reclosed with 0 Ethibond, leaving the cord and nerve in the subcutaneous position. Several sutures of 0 Ethibond were also placed above the emergence of the cord at the internal ring. Subcutaneous tissues were then approximated with 3-0 Vicryl and after irrigation skin was closed with skin clips. The patient tolerated the procedure well and sent to the recovery room in good condition.

PATHOLOGY REPORT—PATIENT 1

DATE SPECIMEN SUBMITTED: 4/5

SPECIMEN: Lipoma of cord

CLINICAL DATA:

GROSS DESCRIPTION: The specimen is submitted as lipoma of cord. It consists of a single irregularly shaped fragment of fatty tissue that is 8.0 × 4.0 × 1.5 cm. It is covered with a thin membrane.

MICROSCOPIC DESCRIPTION:

DIAGNOSIS: Lipomatous tissue of left spermatic cord

PHYSICIAN'S ORDERS—PATIENT 1

DATE	ORDER
4/5	Attending MD: Admit to same-day surgery Betadine scrub ×3 Preop May take own meds
4/5	Anesthesia note: Continue NPO Demerol 50 mg IM 11/2 hr Preop Vistaril 50 mg IM 11/2 hr Preop Atropine 0.4 mg IM 11/2 hr Preop
4/5	Attending MD: Vital signs q. 15 min until stable Regular diet Darvocet-N-100 q. 4 hrs p.r.n. pain Discharge to home when stable

LABORATORY REPORTS—PATIENT 1

HEMATOLOGY

DATE: 4/5

Specimen	Results	Normal Values
WBC	6.83	4.3–11.0
RBC	4.57	4.5–5.9
HGB	13.7	13.5–17.5
HCT	43	41–52
MCV	87.0	80–100
MCHC	35	31–57
PLT	300	150–400

AUTO DIFFERENTIAL

DATE: 4/5

Specimen	Results	Normal Values
NEUT	68.3	40.0–74.0
LYMPH	20	19.0–48.0
MONO	5.6	3.4–9.0
EOS	5.6	0.0–7.0
BASO	0.6	0.0–1.5
LUC	3.8	0.0–4.0

URINALYSIS

DATE: 4/5

Test	Result	Ref Range
SP GRAVITY	1.017	1.005–1.035
PH	6	5–7
PROT	TRACE	NEG
GLUC	NONE	NEG
KETONES	NONE	NEG
BILI	NONE	NEG
BLOOD	TRACE	NEG
NITRATES	NONE	NEG
RBCS	NONE	NEG
WBCS	NONE	NEG

RADIOLOGY REPORT—PATIENT 1

DATE: 4/5

DIAGNOSIS: Inguinal hernia

EXAMINATION: Chest x-ray

Heart size and shape are acceptable. The lung fields are clear and the pulmonary vascular pattern is unremarkable. There is no free fluid and the trachea remains midline.

Enter two diagnosis codes and two procedure codes.

PDX: Direct Ing hernia

DX2: Lipoma spermatic cord

PP1:

PR2:

AMBULATORY CASE—PATIENT 2

DIAGNOSIS: Low back pain, lumbar radiculopathy with chronic pain syndrome

HISTORY: This is an 18-year-old white female with low back pain and lumbar radicular pain for epidural steroid injection. The patient had an epidural approximately three weeks ago with approximately 30% improvement. The patient is agreeable for additional epidural steroid injection for pain management.

PROCEDURE: Epidural steroid injection under C-arm guidance via caudal approach and epidurogram. The patient was transferred to the operating room and placed in the prone position. Under MAC anesthesia her low back and sacral areas were sterilely prepped and draped. Local 1% lidocaine was applied with a #23-gauge needle through the skin and surrounding tissues of the sacral hiatus. Then a #17-gauge Epimed needle was inserted percutaneously through the sacral hiatus into the epidural space. This was confirmed via lateral view of the C-arm. Then under AP fluoroscopy, a #18-gauge Epimed catheter was guided to the mid L3-L4 area of the nerve root in the midline. Next, 2 cc of Isovue dye was injected, which showed good bilateral spread in the epidural space. A solution of 6 cc of normal saline, 80 mg of Depo-Medrol and 2 cc of 1% lidocaine was partially deposited at the L3-L4 nerve root. The catheter was then moved down to the L4-L5 nerve root in the midline of the epidural space. An additional 1 cc of Isovue dye was injected, which showed good bilateral spread. An additional one third of local anesthetic Depo-Medrol solution was deposited at the L4-L5 nerve root. The catheter was then moved down to the L5-S1 nerve root and in the midline. Another 1 cc of Isovue dye was injected, which confirmed good bilateral spread and highlighting of the L5-S1 nerve roots bilateral. The remaining local anesthetic Depo-Medrol solution was deposited at the L5-S1 nerve root. The catheter and needle were then pulled intact and the patient was transferred to the recovery room in satisfactory condition.

IMPRESSION: Low back pain, lumbar radiculopathy. This is the patient's second epidural steroid injection.

FOLLOW-UP: After seeing improvement in the next 24 to 48 hours and repeat injection if necessary.

Enter two diagnosis codes and one procedure code.

PDX

DX2

PP1

AMBULATORY RECORD—PATIENT 3

DATE: 8/12/20XX

SURGERY RECORD:

PATIENT HISTORY: This patient is seen today to insert an intrathecal pump for pain management due to ductal carcinoma of the left upper breast metastatic to the spine. She previously underwent modified radical mastectomy with general anesthesia and had no adverse effects. No other surgical history is given. No known allergies, no current medications. Review of systems is normal ASA = 2.

Following preoperative evaluation and discussion with the patient, local anesthesia was used to implant an intrathecal programmable pump surgically placed and attached to a previously placed catheter. The patient tolerated the procedure well. There were no adverse effects of anesthesia.

AMBULATORY RECORD—PATIENT 3

Enter three diagnosis codes and one procedure code.

PDX	Pain Management
DX2	Met. bone
DX3	CA Brn
PP1	

AMBULATORY RECORD—PATIENT 4

PREOPERATIVE DIAGNOSIS: Reflex sympathetic dystrophy, left knee

POSTOPERATIVE DIAGNOSIS: Reflex sympathetic dystrophy, left knee

OPERATION: Left lumbar sympathetic block with C-arm

ANESTHESIA: Local

INDICATIONS:
This 43-year-old female has a 7-month history of left knee pain. She says that even a light touch appears to be exquisitely painful. She has had surgery to clear scar tissue.

PROCEDURE DESCRIPTION:
The patient was placed on the x-ray lucent gurney in the right lateral decubitus position. The back was prepped with Betadine, and the midline spinous processes were marked. A line was drawn 6 to 7 cm lateral to that midline on the left. L2 was identified using the C-arm and lateral projections, and lidocaine was infiltrated at the skin. The 22-gauge, 6-inch Chiba needle was advanced down to and off the body of L2, and loss of resistance was obtained with a glass syringe. Renografin-60 was injected and showed a good distribution. So 15 cc of bupivacaine 0.5% without epinephrine was injected, plus Depo-Medrol 40 mg. The needle was withdrawn.

Then lidocaine was infiltrated on the 6- to 7-cm line at L4. I advanced the 22-gauge, 6-inch needle off the body of L4, but the Renografin-60 distribution appeared not to be adequate. Another wheal was raised at the 13 level, and the needle was advanced down to and off the body of L3. A loss of resistance was obtained with a glass syringe, followed by Renografin-60. This time, the distribution was excellent, and bupivacaine 0.5% without epinephrine ×15 cc was injected. She was left on her side for 25 minutes. After 10 minutes, she had a noticeably warmer left foot and ankle. The skin coloration of the left leg was normal.

Enter one diagnosis code and two procedure codes.

PDX RSD

PP1

PR2

INPATIENT CASE—PATIENT 5

DATE OF ADMISSION: 1/5 **DATE OF DISCHARGE:** 1/7

DISCHARGE DIAGNOSIS:

1. Adenocarcinoma of the endometrium
2. Hemoperitoneum
3. Postoperative hemorrhage
4. Hemorrhagic shock secondary to blood loss

COURSE IN HOSPITAL: The patient was taken to the operating room on 1/5 where a laparoscopically assisted vaginal hysterectomy was carried out.

At approximately 6:30 p.m. on the same day, I was called back into the hospital's recovery room because the patient was in shock with blood pressure of 80/60 with poor urine output and distended abdomen.

At this point it was decided to do an emergency diagnostic laparoscopy with preoperative diagnosis of postoperative hemorrhage. Bleeders were controlled with hemostatic sutures applied through the laparoscope.

The immediate postoperative course was essentially stormy with urine output maintained at 30 mL/h.

An ultrasound of the abdomen and pelvis was requested on the second postoperative day and this revealed normal renal shadow; no abnormal fluid accumulation in the pelvis or in the abdominal wall. The patient was then transferred to the regular floor on 1/6 after having maintained a satisfactory postoperative course from the second surgical procedure. The Jackson-Pratt drain was removed on 1/7 with closure of the abdominal incision with Steri-strips. The patient remained afebrile. She had been out of bed with good urine output and tolerating house diet. Her activities were increased gradually. Hemoglobin was again checked prior to discharge and was 12.1 g.

The patient was discharged to home on 1/7.

INSTRUCTIONS ON DISCHARGE: Regular diet. Follow up with appointment in my office in 3 days and with a colonoscopy for colon screening in light of family history of colon cancer.

HISTORY AND PHYSICAL EXAMINATION—PATIENT 5

ADMITTED: 1/5

REASON FOR ADMISSION: Vaginal bleeding

HISTORY OF PRESENT ILLNESS: This is a 62-year-old white female, gravida IV, para IV. She states that she has been in good health and has not had any gynecological complaints. During the past year she has had some left lower-quadrant pain and has noted post-coital bleeding. The bleeding has also occurred on and off for several months.

PAST MEDICAL HISTORY: Hypothyroidism due to thyroidectomy many years ago for benign tumor. No other serious illnesses, operations, or hospitalizations. The patient takes Synthroid 0.200 mcg.

ALLERGIES: No known drug or food allergies.

CHRONIC MEDICATIONS: Synthroid 0.200 mcg

FAMILY HISTORY: Her mother died of colon cancer at age 53 years.

SOCIAL HISTORY: The patient is married with four children. She does not drink or smoke.

REVIEW OF SYSTEMS: HEENT essentially negative; wears glasses. Cardiorespiratory; no cough, dyspnea, cyanosis or chest pain. Gastrointestinal; no specific digestive or bowel complaints, with the exception of the non-specific left lower quadrant pain. The patient has no specific urinary complaints. The patient has a low hemoglobin level.

PHYSICAL EXAMINATION:

GENERAL APPEARANCE: Well-developed, well-nourished 62-year-old woman in no acute distress

HEENT: Essentially negative

LUNGS: Clear to P & A

HEART: Regular in force, rate, and rhythm. There are no audible murmurs.

ABDOMEN: No hernia or palpable masses. Abdomen is soft and flat. Peristalsis is normal. There are no areas of tenderness.

GENITALIA: Bimanual examination reveals the external genitalia to be normal. The uterus is of normal size. There are no palpable pelvic masses or tenderness.

RECTAL: Negative

IMPRESSION: Postmenopausal bleeding, possible endometrial carcinoma with blood loss anemia

PLAN: Vaginal hysterectomy

PROGRESS NOTES—PATIENT 5

DATE	NOTE
1/5	The patient is admitted for LAVH because of postmenopausal bleeding. She has also had left lower-quadrant pain. General condition is good.
	Operative Note: Preop: Possible adenocarcinoma of the endometrium Postop: Same, pathology pending Procedure: LAVH Anesthesia: General

FINDINGS: Tubes and ovaries were within normal limits. Uterus is submitted for pathologic examination. Estimated blood loss is 300 CCs. Called back to the RR for decrease in blood pressure and decreased urine output. The patient was found to have abdominal distention as well. The patient was given 3 units of blood and taken back to the operating room for evaluation of postoperative hemorrhage.

OPERATIVE NOTE:

Preop: Postop hemorrhage
Postop: Accidental laceration of epigastric artery, acute blood loss anemia
Procedure: Repair of bleeding vessel via laparoscope
Anesthesia: General
EBL: 1,500 to 2,000 mL of blood
The patient was admitted to the ICU following surgery where we will monitor her progress throughout the night.

1/6	Patient is doing well today. The BP is stable, urine output good–diuresing well, wound clean and dry, healing well. Will transfer her to the surgical floor.
1/7	The patient is stable, offers no complaints. Will discharge to home.

	PHYSICIAN'S ORDERS—PATIENT 5
DATE	**ORDER**
1/5	Admit for LAVH
	Type and cross 4 units of blood, CBC Prepare for vaginal hysterectomy Synthroid 0.200 mcg daily NPO Demerol 75 mg Atropin 0.4 mg preop Postop, transfer patient to ICU D5NSS 125 cc/h Transfuse three units PRBC Demerol 75 mg IM q. 4 hours as need for pain Ancef 500 mg q. 6 hrs ×3 doses CBC q. 4 hrs, Strict I & O
1/6	Transfer to floor; please get patient OOB and provide liquids at bedside
	Continue I & O CBC this a.m. then tomorrow a.m. D/C IV after 6:00 p.m. if stable
1/7	Discharge to home

OPERATIVE REPORT—PATIENT 5

DATE: 1/5

PREOPERATIVE DIAGNOSIS: Possible adenocarcinoma of the endometrium

POSTOPERATIVE DIAGNOSIS: Pending pathology report

OPERATION: Laparoscopic assisted vaginal hysterectomy with pelvic cytology

ANESTHESIA: General

OPERATIVE PROCEDURE: With the patient under satisfactory general anesthesia in the semilithotomy position, she was prepped and draped in the usual fashion for a laparoscopic and vaginal procedure. Through an infraumbilical incision, a Veress needle was inserted to establish a pneumoperitoneum using a high-flow insufflator with CO_2 gas, maintaining 15 mm of pressure. It was then followed by insertion of a 10-mm trocar into the infraumbilical incision, followed by the laparoscope with laparoscopic examination having been done with findings described above.

After transillumination of the abdomen noting vessels, an incision was made in the skin and 12-mm trocars and sleeves were inserted into the right and left lower quadrant.

After having inserted the 12-mm sleeves, an endogauge was inserted into Channel A and levels of the right and left tubo-ovarian ligaments and broad ligaments were measured. An endo-GIA was then inserted into Channel A, followed by endo-GIA of Channel B, amputating the attachments of the tubes and ovaries and the broad ligaments. The remaining attachments of the board ligaments and the round ligaments were picked up with endo-GIA staplers on both sides.

A grasper was then inserted on Channel A, and the bladder reflection was picked up and elevated. It was then opened with endoshears, and using hydrodissection and ultrasonic scalpel, a bladder flap was created by sharp and blunt dissection with the scalpel. The dissection was carried down to the surface of the anterior lip of the cervix, which was noted to be smooth and free of adhesions. This was extended down past the cervicovaginal junction with identification of the tenaculum in the vagina. The grasper was then replaced on the right cornua and traction placed on the uterus, exposing the right cardinal ligaments, which was then placed on traction and using the scalpel probe, skeletonization of the uterine arteries with exposure of the arteries was done automatically.

The peritoneum was then dissected down past the uterosacral ligament insertion. After complete skeletonization of the uterine arteries was done, an endo TA-30 stapler was placed on the uterine arteries and the pedicle was cut off with the scalpel. There were no bleeding points noted.

OPERATIVE REPORT—PATIENT 5

The grasper was then removed and inserted into Channel B, and the left cornua of the uterus was picked up and placed on traction. The left cardinal ligaments and uterine arteries were then picked up and skeletonized, and complete exposure and dissection was done with visualization and identification of the arteries. The fragments of paravesical tissue were dissected off with the scalpel without traumatizing the bladder, which had previously been filled up with methylene blue and no spillage of the dye was noted during dissection of the uterus.

An endo TA-30 was then inserted in Channel A and linear staples were placed on the uterine arteries, on the left uterine artery and the cardinal ligament pedicles. The pedicle was then cut off with the scalpel. A second line of staples was then placed below the first line, taking care not to include the dome of the bladder without entering the vagina, and the pedicle cut off with the scalpel. There was a change in color of the uterus from pink to gray, indicating complete obliteration of blood supply.

The staple lines on the infundibular pelvis ligaments were then inspected and this was found to be adequate. At this time the laparoscopic procedure was temporarily stopped and attention was then paid to the vaginal portion of the procedure, releasing the pneumoperitoneum that had been established for the laparoscopy. The cervix was exposed and picked up on the anterior a posterior lip with Lahey clamps, and a circumscribing incision was made on the cervicovaginal junction down to the level of the paravesical fascia and dissected off by sharp and blunt dissection with entry into the anterior cul-de-sac atraumatically, and the posterior cul-de-sac entered likewise.

The insertions of the base of the uterosacral ligaments and cardinal ligaments were then picked up with Heaney clamps, cut and suture ligated with #0 Vicryl, followed by a second line of Heaney clamps on the base of the remaining portion of the cardinal ligaments that was attached to the uterus, amputating and freeing up the uterus. The pedicles were tied off with #0 Vicryl materials and the uterus pulled and delivered out of the abdominal cavity through the vagina. Angle sutures were then placed on the vaginal cuff using #0 Vicryl material, and the intervening incision was closed with vertical mattress sutures using #0 Vicryl material.

After having closed the vagina and establishing adequate hemostasis, attention was once again placed on the laparoscopic portion. The pneumoperitoneum was once again established using high-flow insufflator and CO_2 gas at 10-mm pressure, and inspection and irrigation of the vascular pedicles and the vaginal cuff was done, which revealed them to be dry. The pelvis was irrigated with copious amounts of warm saline solution. The procedure was then terminated. The sleeve and gripper in Channel A was removed, and was found to be dry. The fascia was closed using an endo close needle with a #0 Vicryl suture in interrupted fashion using three stitches. The channel B 12-mm sheath and trocar were removed, which were dry.

OPERATIVE REPORT—PATIENT 5

At this time, termination of the procedure was done. The laparoscope was removed and the CO_2 released gradually. All instruments were removed and remaining stab wounds were closed in the fascia with #0 Vicryl sutures, and subcutaneously with #4-0 Monocryl. Sterile dressings were applied.

The patient was transferred to the recovery room in a reactive state with stable vital signs. Estimated blood loss was 300 mL of whole blood, no replacement given.

PATHOLOGY REPORT—PATIENT 5

DATE: 1/5

SPECIMEN: Uterus

CLINICAL DATA:

PREOPERATIVE DIAGNOSIS: Adenocarcinoma of endometrium

POSTOPERATIVE DIAGNOSIS: Same

GROSS DESCRIPTION: The specimen is labeled "Uterus." Submitted uterus with cervix attached. The specimen has previously been partially opened. It measures 9 × 5 × 3 cm and weight 58 g. The body of the uterus appears to be symmetrical. On section, the endocervix and ectocervix appear essentially normal. The endocervical canal likewise appears normal. The endometrial cavity is involved by a polypoid tumor mass chiefly in the right cornual area and measuring 3 cm in greatest diameter. The tumor appears to superficially penetrate the myometrium. The specimen will be further sectioned following fixation.

A and B are sections of cervix; C, D, E, F, G, and H are full-thickness section of tumor; section I is a full-thickness section from grossly uninvolved tissue.

MICROSCOPIC DESCRIPTION:

DIAGNOSIS: Adenocarcinoma, intermediate grade, of endometrium. Chronic cervicitis

COMMENT: The tumor penetrates approximately 0.4 cm into a total myometrial thickness of 1.5 cm.

OPERATIVE REPORT—PATIENT 5

DATE: 1/5

PREOPERATIVE DIAGNOSIS: Postoperative hemorrhage

POSTOPERATIVE DIAGNOSIS: Bleeding from right epigastric artery

OPERATION: Emergency diagnostic laparoscopy with repair of epigastric artery and blood transfusion

ANESTHESIA: General

OPERATIVE INDICATIONS: Estimated blood loss 1,500 to 2,000 mL of whole blood

OPERATIVE PROCEDURE: There was liquid and clotted blood in the abdominal cavity, approximately 1,500 to 2,000 mL, with blood coming from the puncture in the right lower quadrant, apparently from an accidental laceration of the right epigastric artery. The pedicles were inspected in the pelvis, and these were found to be dry.

With the patient under satisfactory general anesthesia, after having been transfused three units of packed RBCs, she was taken to the operating room and an emergency laparoscopic examination was carried out by opening the previous stab wounds with irrigation of the abdominal and pelvic cavity, evacuating approximately 1,500 to 2,000 mL of liquid and clotted blood.

Exposure of the pedicles of the infundibulopelvic ligament on both sides and the uterine arteries and the vaginal vault revealed them to be dry. There was no bleeding anywhere else in the pelvic cavity.

A puncture was found in the epigastric artery. Using an endoclosed needle through which a #0 Vicryl ligature was attached, the artery was repaired, stopping the bleeding point. This was verified by inspection with the laparoscope. After this was accomplished, the fascia was once again closed with endoclosed needle and #0 Vicryl suture on the right lower quadrant. The left lower quadrant was left open, and a Jackson-Pratt drain was inserted into the incision and placed in the pelvis for drainage.

The patient was then removed from the Trendelenburg position after ascertaining that vital signs were stable. The CO_2 was released gradually. All instruments were removed, and subcuticular closure of the stab wounds was done using #4-0 Monocryl sutures.

At the termination of surgery the patient's vital signs were stable. She, however, remained hypotensive with tachycardia with good urine output and was transfused an additional three units and transferred to the intensive care unit for postoperative care.

LABORATORY REPORTS—PATIENT 5

HEMATOLOGY

Specimen	Results				Normal Values
	1/5	1/5	1/5	1/7	
WBC	5.0	5.0	5.2	5.1	4.3-11.0
RBC	5.0	4.0 L	4.2 L	4.5	4.5-5.9
HGB	7.1 L	5.5 L	7.9 L	9.0 L	13.5-17.5
HCT	38 L	32 L	39 L	43	41-52
MCV	90	89	97	96	80-100
MCHC	44	46	48	50	31-57
PLT	160	165	170	300	150-400

LABORATORY REPORTS—PATIENT 5

HEMATOLOGY

Specimen	Results				Normal Values
	1/5	1/5	1/6	1/7	
WBC	9.2	9.5	9.8	9.7	4.3-11.0
RBC	4.6	4.8	5.1	5.2	4.5-5.9
HGB	10.1 L	10.3 L	11.0 L	12.1 L	13.5-17.5
HCT	44	41	45	44	41-52
MCV	90	89	97	96	80-100
MCHC	44	46	48	50	31-57
PLT	160	165	170	300	150-400

Enter nine diagnosis codes and two procedure codes.

PDX Aden carc.

DX2 hemoperitoneum

DX3 Postop hem

DX4 Hem. shock due to bloodloss

DX5 blood loss anemia

DX6 Compl. Post op - hemm.

DX7 Ch Cervicitis

DX8 Hemm. epi artery

DX9 Acc laceration

PP1

PR2

CCS
Practice Exam 1

A blank answer sheet for these multiple choice questions can be found on page 85.

Domain 1: Health Information Documentation

1. A 7-year-old patient was admitted to the emergency department for treatment of shortness of breath. The patient is given epinephrine and nebulizer treatments. The shortness of breath and wheezing are unabated following treatment. What diagnosis should be suspected?

   a. Acute bronchitis

   b. Acute bronchitis with chronic obstructive pulmonary disease

   c. Asthma with status asthmaticus

   d. Chronic obstructive asthma

2. A patient is admitted with a high temperature, lethargy, hypotension, tachycardia, oliguria, and elevated WBC. The patient also has more than 100,000 organisms of *Escherichia coli* per cc of urine. The attending physician documents "urosepsis." What is the next step for the coder?

   a. Code sepsis as the principal with a secondary diagnosis of urinary tract infection due to *E. coli.*

   b. Code urinary tract infection with sepsis as a secondary diagnosis.

   c. Query the physician to determine if the patient is being treated for sepsis, highlighting the clinical signs and symptoms.

   d. Ask the physician whether the patient had septic shock so that this may be used as the principal diagnosis.

3. During a coronary artery bypass surgery, the patient underwent saphenous bypass grafts; from the aorta to the left anterior descending branch of the left main coronary artery, and the left posterior descending of the left main coronary artery. The patient also underwent a repositioning of the mammary artery to the right coronary artery. Choose the best description for this procedure.

   a. Three aortocoronary grafts

   b. Two aortocoronary grafts and one mammary-coronary graft

   c. Two aortocoronary grafts and two saphenous bypass graft

   d. Three aortocoronary grafts and one mammary-coronary graft

4. According to CPT, an endoscopy that is undertaken to the level of the midtransverse colon would be coded as a:

   a. Proctosigmoidoscopy

   b. Sigmoidoscopy

   c. Colonoscopy

   d. Proctoscopy

5. Infusion of Herceptin which is a monoclonal antibody used for treatment of breast cancer in patients carrying a certain mutation of the HER2 gene is classified as:
   a. Chemotherapy
   b. Radiotherapy
   c. Genotherapy
   d. Immunotherapy

6. A patient has findings suggestive of chronic obstructive pulmonary disease (COPD) on chest x-ray. The attending physician mentions the x-ray finding in one progress note but no medication, treatment, or further evaluation is provided. The coder should:
   a. Query the attending physician regarding the x-ray finding.
   b. Code the condition because the documentation reflects it.
   c. Question the radiologist regarding whether to code this condition.
   d. Use a code from abnormal findings to reflect the condition.

7. If a patient undergoes an inpatient procedure and the final summary diagnosis is different from the diagnosis on the pathology report, the coder should:
   a. Code only from the discharge diagnoses.
   b. Code the diagnosis reflected on the pathology report.
   c. Code the most severe symptom.
   d. Query the attending physician as to the final diagnosis.

8. A 56-year-old woman is admitted to an acute-care facility from a skilled nursing facility. The patient has multiple sclerosis and hypertension. During the course of hospitalization a decubitus ulcer is found and debrided at the bedside by a physician. There is no typed operative report and no pathology report. The coder should:
   a. Use an excisional debridement code as these charts are rarely reviewed to verify the excisional debridement.
   b. Code with a nonexcisional debridement procedure code.
   c. Query the healthcare provider who performed the procedure to determine if the debridement was excisional.
   d. Eliminate the procedure code all together.

9. A 23-year-old female is admitted for shock following treatment of a miscarriage. The pathology report from the previous admission reveals that the patient had no decidua or products of conception in the tissue removed. This encounter would be coded as:

   a. 634, Spontaneous abortion

   b. 639, Complication following abortion and ectopic and molar pregnancies

   c. 785.50, Shock NOS

   d. 998.0, Postoperative shock

Domain 2: Diagnosis Coding

10. A patient is admitted for chest pain and new onset angina was diagnosed. The patient was stabilized and discharged. In a subsequent admission, the patient was admitted as an outpatient for a left heart catheterization, coronary arteriography using two catheters and left ventricular angiography. The patient was found to have arteriosclerotic heart disease. The angina is controlled with medication and the patient has no history of cardiac surgery. The appropriate sequencing of ICD-9 and CPT codes for the outpatient catheterization would be:

411.1	Intermediate coronary syndrome (Unstable angina)
413.9	Other and unspecified angina pectoris
414.00	Coronary atherosclerosis of unspecified type of vessel, native or graft
414.01	Coronary atherosclerosis of native coronary artery
786.50	Chest pain, unspecified
93452	Left heart catheterization including intraprocedural injection(s) for left ventriculography, imaging supervision and interpretation, when performed
93453	Combined right and left heart catheterization including intraprocedureal injection(s) for left ventriculography, imaging supervision and interpretation, when performed
93454	Catheter placement in coronary artery(s) for coronary angiography, including intraprocedural injection(s) for coronary angiography, imaging supervision and interpretation
93458	with left heart catheterization including intraprocedural injection(s) for left ventriculography, when performed

   a. 786.50, 93452

   b. 411.1, 93510, 93454

   c. 414.01, 413.9, 93453

   d. 414.01, 93458

11. A 65-year-old patient is admitted with pain and loosening of a previous total hip arthroplasty. The acetabular component has loosened and become painful. The patient was admitted for revision of the hip replacement. The acetabular component uses a metal-on-metal bearing surface. What is the appropriate code(s) for the admission?

996.41	Mechanical loosening of prosthetic joint
996.66	Infection and inflammatory reaction due to internal joint prosthesis
V43.64	Organ or tissue replaced by other means, hip
00.71	Revision of hip replacement, acetabular component
00.74	Hip-bearing surface, metal on polyethylene
00.75	Hip-bearing surface, metal on metal
00.76	Hip-bearing surface, ceramic on ceramic

a. 996.41, V43.64, 00.71, 00.75

b. 996.66, 00.75

c. 996.41, V43.64, 00.71

d. 996.66, V43.64, 00.71, 00.75

12. A maternity patient is admitted in labor at 43 weeks. She has a normal delivery with vacuum extraction to facilitate the baby's delivery. Which of the following would be the principal diagnosis?

650	Normal delivery
645.11	Post-term pregnancy, delivered, with or without mention of antepartum condition
645.21	Prolonged pregnancy, delivered, with or without mention of antepartum condition
669.51	Forceps or vacuum extractor delivery without mention of indication, delivered, with or without mention of antepartum condition

a. 645.11

b. 645.21

c. 650

d. 669.51

13. With regard to the implementation of ICD-10-CM, all of the following are correct except?

a. ICD-10-CM was developed by NCHS

b. ICD-10-CM and ICD-10-PCS will be fully implemented beginning October 1, 2012

c. ICD-10 is already being used in the United States for death certificate coding

d. The process of adoption of ICD-10-CM is specified in HIPAA

14. A 75-year-old female was admitted for acute myocardial infarction and underwent a diagnostic cardiac catheterization. Following the catheterization, the patient developed a pseudoaneurysm documented as due to the catheterization in the common femoral artery. The pseudoaneurysm would be coded as:

    a. 997.2, Peripheral vascular complication
       442.3, Other aneurysm of artery of lower extremity

    b. 998.2, Accidental puncture or laceration during a procedure
       442.3, Other aneurysm of artery of lower extremity

    c. 442.3, Other aneurysm of artery of lower extremity

    d. 998.2, Accidental puncture or laceration during a procedure

15. A patient was admitted to the emergency department with chest pain, and was diagnosed with aborted myocardial infarction with acute myocardial ischemia. There was no prior cardiac surgery. The cardiac enzymes were normal. The appropriate coding of the diagnosis for this case is:

    a. 410.91, Acute myocardial infarction, unspecified site

    b. 414.01, Coronary atherosclerosis of native coronary artery

    c. 411.89, Other acute and subacute forms of ischemic heart disease

    d. 411.81, Acute coronary occlusion without myocardial infarction

16. A patient has nausea and vomiting with abdominal pain due to acute cholecystitis. The physician documents the following on the discharge summary: acute cholecystitis, nausea, vomiting, and abdominal pain. The diagnosis(es) that would be coded is(are):

    a. Acute cholecystitis, nausea, vomiting, and abdominal pain

    b. Acute cholecystitis, nausea, vomiting

    c. Acute cholecystitis, nausea

    d. Acute cholecystitis

17. A patient is admitted because of congestive heart failure (CHF). During the treatment of the CHF the patient was also found to have elevated liver function tests. The physician worked-up the elevated liver function tests but was not able to determine a diagnosis with regard to the abnormal liver tests. The coder should identify the following diagnosis(es) when coding the record:

    a. Congestive heart failure with liver disease

    b. Abnormal liver function tests

    c. Congestive heart failure and a code from the findings abnormal section

    d. Congestive heart failure

18. A patient is admitted with hypotension due to dobutamine taken, administered, and prescribed correctly. How should this be coded?

    a. 458.0, Orthostatic hypotension
    E941.2, Adverse effects of dobutamine

    b. 458.29, Other iatrogenic hypotension
    E941.2, Adverse effects of dobutamine

    c. 458.8, Other specified hypotension
    E941.2, Adverse effects of dobutamine

    d. 458.1, Chronic hypotension
    E941.2, Adverse effects of dobutamine

19. A patient is readmitted two weeks after a laminectomy for spinal stenosis due to a defect in the dura. The patient is taken to the operating room for repair of the dura. The code(s) assigned for this admission would be:

    a. 724.02, Spinal stenosis, lumbar region, without neurogenic claudication

    b. 349.31, Accidental puncture or laceration of dura during a procedure
    349.0 Spinal fluid loss headache

    c. 952.2, Laceration of dura

    d. 724.02, Spinal stenosis, lumbar region, without neurogenic claudication
    952.2, Laceration of dura

20. A patient is admitted to the hospital with shortness of breath and congestive heart failure and subsequently develops respiratory failure. The patient undergoes intubation with ventilator management. The correct coding and sequencing of the diagnoses in this case would be:

    a. Congestive heart failure, respiratory failure, ventilator management, intubation

    b. Respiratory failure, intubation, ventilator management

    c. Respiratory failure, congestive heart failure, intubation, ventilator management

    d. Shortness of breath, congestive heart failure, respiratory failure, ventilator management, intubation

21. If a patient is admitted with pneumococcal pneumonia and pneumococcal sepsis, the coder should:

    a. Assign a code for only the sepsis and pneumonia.

    b. Assign a code for the sepsis, pneumonia, and SIRS.

    c. Assign only a code for pneumococcal pneumonia.

    d. Review the chart to determine if septic shock could be used first.

22. A patient was admitted with end stage renal disease (ESRD) following kidney transplant. The patient also had angina and chronic obstructive pulmonary disease. The diagnoses would be coded and sequenced as:
    a. Kidney failure; status post kidney transplant; chronic obstructive pulmonary disease; angina
    b. End-stage renal disease; status post kidney transplant; chronic obstructive pulmonary disease; angina
    c. Chronic kidney disease, stage V; status post kidney transplant; chronic obstructive pulmonary disease; angina
    d. Acute kidney failure; status post kidney transplant; chronic obstructive pulmonary disease; angina

Domain 3: Procedure Coding

23. Which of the following is *not* part of a facility coding compliance plan?
    a. Regular internal audits
    b. Audits performed by objective external reviewers
    c. Coding audits performed by payers
    d. Sharing and discussing results with coding staff

24. In CPT, unlisted codes are reported only if:
    a. There is not a current CPT category I code available
    b. There is not a current CPT category III code available
    c. There is not a current CPT category II code available
    d. There is not a current CPT category I or III code available

25. A virtual screening colonoscopy would be coded as:

45378	Colonoscopy, flexible, proximal to splenic flexure; diagnostic, with or without collection of specimen(s) by brushing or washing, with or without colon decompression (separate procedure)
45391	Colonoscopy, flexible, proximal to splenic flexure; with endoscopic ultrasound examination
74263	Computed tomographic (CT) colonography, screening, including including image postprocessing.
76376	3D rendering with interpretation and reporting of computed tomography, magnetic resonance imaging, ultrasound, or other tomographic modality, not requiring image postprocessing on an independent workstation

a. 74263

b. 45391

c. 45378

d. 76376

26. A patient underwent an excision of a malignant lesion of the chest that measured 1.0 cm and there was a 0.2 cm margin on both sides. Based on the 2011 CPT codes, which code would be used for the procedure?

a. 11401, Excision benign lesion of trunk . . . excised diameter 0.6 cm to 1.0 cm

b. 11601, Excision malignant lesion of trunk . . . excised diameter 0.6 cm to 1.0 cm

c. 11602, Excision malignant lesion of trunk . . . excised diameter 1.1 cm to 2.0 cm

d. 11402, Excision benign lesion of trunk . . . excised diameter 1.1 cm to 2.0 cm

27. A patient was diagnosed with L4-5 lumbar neuropathy and discogenic pain. The patient underwent an intradiscal electrothermal annuloplasty (IDET) in the radiology suite. What ICD-9-CM code should be used?

a. 80.50, Excision, destruction and other repair of intervertebral disc, unspecified

b. 04.2, Destruction of cranial and peripheral nerves

c. 80.59, Other destruction of intervertebral disc

d. 05.23, Lumbar sympathectomy

28. A laparoscopic tubal ligation with Falope ring is completed. What is the correct CPT code assignment?

49321	Laparoscopy, surgical; with biopsy (single or multiple)
58662	Laparoscopy, surgical; with fulguration or excision of lesions of the ovary, pelvic viscera, or peritoneal surface by any method
58670	Laparoscopy, surgical; with fulguration of oviducts (with or without transection)
58671	Laparoscopy, surgical; with occlusion of oviducts by device (eg, band, clip, or Falope ring)

a. 49321, 58662

b. 58670

c. 58671

d. 49321

29. Carcinoma of multiple overlapping sites of the bladder. Diagnostic cystoscopy and transurethral fulguration of bladder lesions (1.9 cm, 6.0 cm) are undertaken. The appropriate CPT code(s) would be:

52000	Cystourethroscopy
52224	Cystourethroscopy, with fulguration (including cryosurgery or laser surgery) or treatment of minor (less than 0.5 cm) lesion(s) with or without biopsy
52234	Cystourethroscopy, with fulguration (including cryosurgery or laser surgery) and/or resection of small bladder tumor(s) (0.5 cm to 2.0 cm)
52235	Cystourethroscopy, with fulguration (including cryosurgery or laser surgery) and/or resection of medium bladder tumor(s) (2.0 cm to 5.0 cm)
52240	Cystourethroscopy, with fulguration (including cryosurgery or laser surgery) and/or resection of large bladder tumor(s)

a. 52234, 52240

b. 52235

c. 52240

d. 52000, 52234, 52260

30. A patient presents to a facility for upper endoscopy implant of material into the muscle of the lower esophageal sphincter. The correct coding and sequencing of this patient's record is:

43235	Upper gastrointestinal endoscopy including esophagus, stomach, and either the duodenum and/or jejunum as appropriate; diagnostic, with or without collection of specimen(s) by brushing or washing (separate procedure)
43257	with delivery of thermal energy to the muscle of lower esophageal sphincter and/or gastric cardia, for treatment of gastroesophageal reflux disease
43258	with ablation of tumor(s) polyp(s), or other lesion(s) not amenable to removal by hot biopsy forceps, bipolar cautery or snare technique
43236	with directed submucosal injection(s), any substance
-59	Distinct procedure service

a. 43257

b. 43235, 43236

c. 43236

d. 43258, 43236–59

31. A patient undergoes a colposcopy with endometrial biopsy. Which of the following is correct?

a. The colposcopy and endometrial biopsy are represented by a combination code.

b. Two codes would be used with modifier –59 appended.

c. Two codes would be used in accordance with 2011 CPT code revisions.

d. Only one code is used and it does not state that it includes endometrial biopsy specifically.

32. A patient presents to the outpatient surgical area for a cystoscopy with multiple biopsies of the bladder. The patient's presenting symptom is hematuria. What is the correct code assignment for this procedure?

52000	Cystourethroscopy (separate procedure)
52204	Cystourethroscopy with biopsy(s)
-22	Increased procedural services

a. 52000

b. 52000–22

c. 52204

d. 52204–22

33. If a patient has an excision of a malignant lesion of the skin, the CPT code is determined by the body area from which the excision occurs and the:

    a. Length of the lesion as described in the pathology report

    b. Dimension of the specimen submitted as described in the pathology report

    c. Width times the length of the lesion as described in the operative report

    d. Diameter of the lesion as well as the margins excised as described in the operative report

Domain 4: Regulatory Guidelines and Reporting Requirements for Acute-Care (Inpatient) Service

34. Documentation in the record reveals that a patient is admitted with an acute exacerbation of COPD (MS-DRG 192). A higher-paying DRG may be appropriate if documentation is present in the record at the time the decision was made to admit the patient that confirms a diagnosis associated with which of the following:

    a. Angina was treated with nitroglycerin prn for chest pain

    b. Atrial fibrillation and underwent a cardioversion while hospitalized

    c. Blood gases of pO_2 of 58, pCO_2 of 55, pH of 7.32 upon admission and treated with intubation and mechanical ventilation for more than 96 hours

    d. Anemia and was given a blood transfusion

35. A female patient is diagnosed with congestive heart failure. Which of the following will optimize the MS-DRG if present on admission?

    a. Atrial fibrillation

    b. Stage III pressure ulcer

    c. Blood loss anemia

    d. Coronary artery disease

36. If the principal diagnosis is an initial episode of an anterior wall myocardial infarction, which procedure will result in the highest DRG?

    a. Mechanical ventilator

    b. Insertion central venous catheter

    c. Right heart cardiac catheterization

    d. Transbronchial lung biopsy

37. Patient admitted with hemorrhage due to placenta previa with twin pregnancy. This patient had two prior (cesarean section) deliveries. Emergent C-section delivery was performed due to the hemorrhage. The appropriate principal diagnosis would be:

    a. Prior cesarean sections

    b. Placenta previa without hemorrhage

    c. Twin gestation

    d. Placenta previa with hemorrhage

38. A patient is admitted with spotting and fever. She is found to have been treated for a miscarriage (spontaneous abortion), which was resolved two weeks prior to this admission. She is treated with aspiration dilation and curettage and products of conception are found. She is found to be septic. Which of the following should be the principal diagnosis?

    a. Complications following abortion and ectopic and other pregnancy

    b. Complications of spontaneous abortion with sepsis

    c. Sepsis

    d. Incomplete spontaneous abortion with sepsis

39. A patient is admitted with an acute inferior myocardial infarction and discharged alive. Which condition would optimize the DRG?

    a. Respiratory failure

    b. Atrial fibrillation

    c. Hypertension

    d. History of myocardial infarction

Domain 5: Regulatory Guidelines and Reporting Requirements for Outpatient Services

Use the information in this table to answer questions 40 through 42.

Billing Number	Status Indicator	CPT/HCPCS	APC*
989323	V	99285-25	00616
989323	T	25500	00129
989323	X	72050	00261
989323	S	72128	08005
989323	N	70450	19937

**This is not the actual reimbursement for the designated APC.*

40. From the information provided, how many APCs would impact this patient's total reimbursement?
    a. 1
    b. 5
    c. 4
    d. Unable to determine

41. What percentage will the facility be paid for procedure code 25500?
    a. 50%
    b. 75%
    c. 0%
    d. 100%

42. If another status T procedure were performed, how much would the facility receive for the second status T procedure?
    a. 50%
    b. 75%
    c. 0%
    d. 100%

43. When a Medicare patient receives an injection of IM penicillin G benzathine, 1,000,000 units only, what is the appropriate code assignment?

96372	Therapeutic, prophylactic or diagnostic injection (specify substance or drug); subcutaneous or intramuscular
96374	Therapeutic, prophylactic or diagnostic injection (specify substance or drug); intravenous push, single or initial substance/drug
J0570	Injection, penicillin G benzathine, up to 1,200,000 units
J0580	Injection, penicillin G benzathine, up to 2,400,000 units

a. 96372

b. J0580

c. 96374

d. 96372, J0570

44. Determining medical necessity for outpatient services includes all the following except:

a. Local coverage determinations (LCDs)

b. National coverage determinations (NCDs)

c. Diagnoses linked to procedures by claims-processing software tests ensuring that the procedure is cross-referenced, or linked, correctly to an acceptable diagnosis code for that service

d. Requiring new HCPCS Codes be developed to replace codes in the CPT codebook

45. According to the UHDDS, section III, the definition of *other diagnoses* is all conditions that:

a. Coexist at the time of admission, that develop subsequently, or that affect the treatment received and/or the length of stay.

b. Receive evaluation and is documented by the physician

c. Receive clinical evaluation, therapeutic treatment, further evaluation, extend the length of stay, increase nursing monitoring/care

d. Are considered to be essential by the physicians involved and are reflected in the record

Domain 6: Data Quality and Management

46. The outpatient code editor (OCE) has all of the following types of edits except:
    a. Claim accuracy
    b. Discharge date discrepancy
    c. Assigning APCs to the claim
    d. Age and sex edits

Refer to the following data when answering questions 47and 48. (*Note:* The DRG weights are not actual weights for fiscal year 2011.)

MS-DRG	MS-DRG Weight	Number of Patients
MS-DRG 193, Simple pneumonia and pleurisy age >17 w/ CC	3.0	10
MS-DRG 195, Simple pneumonia without MCC or CC	2.0	10
MS-DRG 192, Chronic obstructive pulmonary disease w/o CC	1.0	10

47. The case-mix index for the information provided above is:
    a. 0.679
    b. 0.89
    c. 2.0
    d. 0.75

48. The information provided shows that:
    a. The payment is higher for patients with pneumonia with CCs than without.
    b. There are more patients with pneumonia without MCCs than with MCCs.
    c. There is a large pediatric population at this hospital with pneumonia.
    d. There is inaccurate coding of pneumonia at this institution.

49. A nurse inadvertently recorded an incorrect vital sign in a patient electronic health record. The next day, a correction was made in the electronic health record. This resulted in the corrected vital sign being recorded at the time the correction was made due to the software. What would be the result of this correction?
    a. The vital signs would be listed in the correct sequence.
    b. When a correction is made in an electronic health record, the incorrect data is deleted.
    c. The quality of patient care would not be affected.
    d. There was a distorted trend line of vital signs data.

50. According to the UHDDS, in order to assign a code for another diagnosis, documentation must be present that:
    a. The condition is recorded in the patient record by a dietary clerk.
    b. The condition is present in the admission department data.
    c. The condition was clinically evaluated or therapeutically treated, extended the length of hospital stay or increased nursing care and/or monitoring or care.
    d. The condition is considered to be essential by the family.

Domain 7: Information and Communication Technologies

51. Data warehousing to form clinical repositories is undertaken by merging insurance members' claims and clinical data. Data mining assists in all of the following *except:*
    a. Cost cutting
    b. Suggest more appropriate medical treatments
    c. Providing feedback to patients
    d. Predict medical outcomes

52. DRG and APC groupers are usually part of an encoding system in which of the following healthcare settings?
    a. Physician offices
    b. Long-term care facilities
    c. Acute-care hospitals
    d. Outpatient clinics

53. Data, people, and processes along with a combination of hardware, software, and communications technology are components of a(n):
    a. Information system
    b. Classification system
    c. Operating system
    d. Security information

Domain 8: Privacy, Confidentiality, Legal, and Ethical Issues

54. Based on the AHIMA Code of Ethics, which of the following is *not* considered an ethical activity?

    a. Coding audits

    b. Educational purposes within the department

    c. Reviewing the history and physical of a coworker when not part of work assignment

    d. Completion of code assignment

55. Retention policies for the health information department depend on organizational retention policies that must be in accordance with local, state, and federal laws and regulations. These policies vary from institution to institution. In many instances, healthcare institutions may retain health records longer than the law requires. Which of the following statements best describes how the retention of records should be determined?

    a. Unless state or federal law requires longer periods of time, specific patient health information should be retained for established minimum time periods.

    b. AHIMA has published specific guidelines for retention of health information and these guidelines should be followed for records retention.

    c. The Joint Commission has developed standards for retention of health information which must be followed to maintain accreditation and these standards should be adhered to according to these guidelines with regard to time frames.

    d. Health records should be retained according to their use in a facility and the state and federal laws do not apply to the retention of this health information.

56. A patient is admitted to undergo a laparoscopic cholecystectomy. Following the insertion of the laparoscope into the abdominal cavity, the patient experienced a cardiac arrhythmia and the procedure was terminated. The patient experienced a potentially compensable event resulting in an incident report. Which department may request to see the patient's record?

    a. Pediatrics

    b. Risk Management

    c. Surgical Supply

    d. Dietary Services

Domain 9: Compliance

57. Coding compliance policies should include:
    a. Facility-specific documentation requirements
    b. Payer denials
    c. Schedules for record retention
    d. Suggested codes for optimizing reimbursement

58. Under HIPAA Standards for Code Sets, the sets of codes used to encode the diagnoses and procedures, data elements, and medical concepts must be used in:
    a. Paper claims only
    b. Electronic claims only
    c. Outpatient claims only
    d. Inpatient claims only

59. A patient has an inpatient discharge with principal diagnosis of shoulder pain due to peptic ulcer versus cholecystitis documented on the history and physical. Both are equally treated and well documented. A coder should:
    a. Code whichever diagnosis pays more, if both are equally treated
    b. Use a code from the Findings Abnormal category
    c. Code to the most severe symptom
    d. Code shoulder pain, peptic ulcer, cholecystitis

60. A 75-year-old woman is admitted to the hospital after tripping and falling at home. She underwent an open reduction with internal fixation of the femur. Which of the following would be important to capture in addition to diagnostic codes?
    a. E codes for Cause of Injury and Place of Occurrence
    b. E codes for Cause of Injury, Place of Occurrence, Activity, and Status
    c. E codes for Cause of Injury, Place of Occurrence, and Activity
    d. E codes for Cause of Injury only

Multiple Choice Practice Exam 1 Answers

1. ______	21. ______	41. ______
2. ______	22. ______	42. ______
3. ______	23. ______	43. ______
4. ______	24. ______	44. ______
5. ______	25. ______	45. ______
6. ______	26. ______	46. ______
7. ______	27. ______	47. ______
8. ______	28. ______	48. ______
9. ______	29. ______	49. ______
10. ______	30. ______	50. ______
11. ______	31. ______	51. ______
12. ______	32. ______	52. ______
13. ______	33. ______	53. ______
14. ______	34. ______	54. ______
15. ______	35. ______	55. ______
16. ______	36. ______	56. ______
17. ______	37. ______	57. ______
18. ______	38. ______	58. ______
19. ______	39. ______	59. ______
20. ______	40. ______	60. ______

CCS
Practice Exam 1
Case Studies

Note: Review the Coding Instructions (for the Exam) in the Introduction of this book.

SAME DAY SURGERY SUMMARY

HISTORY AND PHYSICAL EXAMINATION—PATIENT 1

REASON FOR ADMISSION: Breast mass

HISTORY OF PRESENT ILLNESS: The patient is a 57-year-old woman who had a routine mammogram performed last week. A lump was noted on the mammogram about 1.2 cm in size. The patient was referred to me. After an explanation to the patient about the condition, a needle localization breast biopsy was performed which revealed intraductal carcinoma in situ.

PAST MEDICAL HISTORY: Noncontributory

ALLERGIES: None known

CHRONIC MEDICATIONS: None

SOCIAL HISTORY: The patient is a 57-year-old female who is married and lives with her husband. She is a nondrinker and a nonsmoker.

REVIEW OF SYSTEMS: The patient has normal bowels. There is no hematuria or dysuria. The patient has had two colds in the past 6 weeks. She states that she has been having some difficulty sleeping because of worry over this beast mass.

PHYSICAL EXAMINATION: This is a well-developed, well-nourished 57-year-old female who appears younger than her stated age.

HEENT: PERRLA with supple neck

LUNGS: The lungs are clear to percussion and auscultation.

CHEST: The heart has normal rhythm and pulse. There is a mass in the right breast.

ABDOMEN: Abdomen reveals no masses; bowel sounds are heard

EXTREMITIES: Extremities reveal no edema

IMPRESSION: Intraductal carcinoma right breast

PLAN: The patient came back to the office yesterday morning with her husband. The situation was explained to them. Since this is an intraductal carcinoma in situ. Lumpectomy will be performed and sentinel node dissection will be carried out. Whether the patient needs further treatment or not depends on the findings of the permanent sections of the specimen. The patient and her husband understand the situation very well and agreed to proceed with surgery.

OPERATIVE REPORT—PATIENT 1

PREOPERATIVE DIAGNOSIS: Intraductal carcinoma in situ, right breast, status post biopsy

POSTOPERATIVE DIAGNOSIS: Intraductal carcinoma in situ, right breast, status post biopsy

OPERATION: Lumpectomy and sentinel axillary lymph node dissection

ANESTHESIA: General anesthesia with laryngeal intubation

PROCEDURE: After obtaining the informed consent, the patient was brought into the operating room and placed on the table in the supine position. General anesthesia with laryngeal intubation was conducted smoothly. The skin over the right chest and right arm was prepped and draped in the usual sterile manner. The intended incision line was marked with a marking pen. The blue dye for the sentinel node dissection was injected. The breast tissue was massaged. Five minutes were then allowed to pass before the incision was made.

The incision was made with excision of the previous incisional scar. The lymphatics were identified and dissected. The suspicious axillary sentinel nodes were dissected. Then the lumpectomy was performed with upper and lower skin flaps. The dissection of the breast tissue and subcutaneous tissue to raise the two flaps was conducted smoothly. A large lump was dissected and the dissection carried to the pectoralis muscles. The big lump was removed completely. Hemostasis was confirmed by cauterization. The wound was then irrigated with copious amounts of warm water solution. The specimen was sent to pathology and the sentinel nodes were sent separately to pathology. The wound was then closed in layers using 2-0 Vicryl for the deeper layer, 3-0 Vicryl for the subcutaneous tissue, and 4-0 Vicryl for the skin.

The patient tolerated the whole procedure very well and was sent to the recovery room in stable condition after extubation.

Blood loss was minimal. Sponge and needle counts were correct. No drain was left. The specimens were sent to pathology.

PATHOLOGY REPORT—PATIENT 1

DATE: 8/3

SPECIMEN: Breast lump and lymph node

GROSS DESCRIPTION: The specimen is submitted as breast and lymphatic tissue. It consists of breast tissue measuring 2.0 cm, 1.5 cm, 1.0 cm.

DIAGNOSIS: Intraductal carcinoma in situ

Enter one diagnosis code and two procedure codes.

PDX ____________________

PP1 ____________________

PR2 ____________________

SAME DAY SURGERY SUMMARY—PATIENT 2

DATE OF ADMISSION: 8/3 **DATE OF DISCHARGE:** 8/3

DISCHARGE DIAGNOSIS:

1. Sinus infection
2. Chronic otitis media
3. Adenoid hypertrophy

PROCEDURES:

1. Adenoidectomy
2. Bilateral myringotomy

INSTRUCTIONS ON DISCHARGE:

Contact my office for follow-up in 1 week

Take Augmentin 500 mg by mouth BID per day for 10 days

Darvocet 1 tablet every 4 hours for pain as needed

HISTORY AND PHYSICAL EXAMINATION—PATIENT 2

ADMITTED: 8/3

REASON FOR ADMISSION: This is a 35-year-old patient who has recurrent sinusitis and chronic otitis media. The patient also suffers from adenoidal obstruction of the eustachian tubes and nasopharynx. Treatment has consisted of antihistamines and decongestants as well as antibiotic therapy. This has been ineffective to control the inflammation. The patient has requested surgery for definitive treatment of the condition.

PAST MEDICAL HISTORY: Negative

ALLERGIES: None known

CHRONIC MEDICATIONS: None

FAMILY HISTORY: Noncontributory

REVIEW OF SYSTEMS: The patient has had repeated office visits over the past 3 years for sinusitis and otitis media. The patient has no other health problems.

PHYSICAL EXAMINATION: This is a Hispanic female in no acute distress. BP is 120/70. Temp. is 99.0 degrees. Pulse is 72. Respirations 12.

HEENT: Tympanic membranes are red with perforation of the tympanic membrane and hearing loss. Otherwise normal.

NECK: Supple

CHEST: Clear to percussion and auscultation

HEART: Regular force, rate, and rhythm

ABDOMINAL: Normal, no masses

EXTREMITIES: No edema, normal

IMPRESSION: Sinus infection and chronic otitis media

PROGRESS NOTES—PATIENT 2

DATE	NOTE
8/3	Patient is alert and oriented. Admitted to Same Day Surgery for adenoidectomy and insertion of myringotomy tubes.

PREOPERATIVE DIAGNOSIS:
Chronic sinusitis
POSTOPERATIVE DIAGNOSIS:
1. Chronic sinusitis
2. Otitis media; Adenoid obstruction of the eustachian tube and nasopharynx
OPERATION:
Bilateral myringotomy with insertion of Shepard tympanostomy tubes; Adenoidectomy
ANESTHESIA: General
COMPLICATIONS: None
The patient tolerated the procedure well. No bleeding noted. Will discharge patient when transportation available.

PHYSICIAN'S ORDERS—PATIENT 2

DATE	ORDER
8/3	Patient is admitted for adenoidectomy and myringotomy
	Prep patient for surgery
	NPO
	PREOP ORDERS
	Morphine 10 mg IM upon admission
	Atropine 0.4 mg IM upon admission
	POSTOP ORDERS
	Ice collar
	T & A Precautions
	OOB ad lib
	Darvocet-N tabs, one every 4 hours p.r.n. pain
	Demerol 75 mg PO now
	Discharge after 4:00 p.m. when stable

OPERATIVE REPORT—PATIENT 2

DATE: 8/3

PREOPERATIVE DIAGNOSIS: Chronic sinusitis, otitis media, adenoid obstruction of the eustachian tubes and nasopharynx

POSTOPERATIVE DIAGNOSIS: Chronic sinusitis, serous otitis media, adenoid obstruction of the eustachian tubes and nasopharynx

OPERATION: Bilateral myringotomy with insertion of Shepard tympanostomy tubes; Adenoidectomy

ANESTHESIA: General

OPERATIVE PROCEDURE: Following the induction of general anesthesia, patient was prepped and draped in the usual sterile manner for the above mentioned procedures. The left ear was approached first.

The tympanic membrane was found to be injected, retracted, and full of a serous fluid. An anterior myringotomy incision was performed, and a Shepard tympanostomy tube was inserted in place.

Following this, an identical procedure was done on the right side, except on the right side the fluid was gray and viscous, and the tympanic membrane had already developed tympanosclerotic scar tissue throughout the tympanic membrane. An anterior myringotomy incision was performed, and a Shepard tympanostomy tube was inserted in place.

Following this, the patient was prepared and draped in the usual manner for adenoidectomy. With the soft palate retracted, an adenoid mass filling the entire nasopharynx was visualized. It was removed with adenoid curets until the normal anatomical structures of the torus tubarius and the posterior choanae of the nasal passages could clearly be seen. The adenoid tissue trailed into the nose and into the area of the infundibulum of the middle meatus. Hemostasis was achieved.

The patient was awakened from anesthesia and taken to the recovery room in good condition.

PATHOLOGY REPORT—PATIENT 2

DATE: 8/3

SPECIMEN: Adenoids

GROSS DESCRIPTION: The specimen is submitted as adenoids. It consists of multiple fragments of adenoid tissue, the largest measuring 2.5 cm, 1.5 cm, 1.0 cm. These fragments are similar to tonsillar tissues.

MICROSCOPIC DESCRIPTION: There are no significant pathologic lesions seen grossly.

DIAGNOSIS: Adenoids

Enter three diagnosis codes and two procedure codes.

PDX ______________________

DX2 ______________________

DX2 ______________________

PP1 ______________________

PR2 ______________________

SAME DAY SURGERY SUMMARY—PATIENT 3
HISTORY AND PHYSICAL EXAMINATION—PATIENT 3

DATE: 1/29

HISTORY OF PRESENT ILLNESS: This is a 62-year-old gentleman with progressive painful blurring of vision due to aphakic bullous keratopathy with glaucoma. He has undergone previous Molteno implant with poor vision and pain due to ruptured bulla. The patient is admitted for transplant, vitrectomy and lens implantation at this time.

PAST MEDICAL HISTORY: The patient has angina and COPD. There have been no recent episodes of chest pain or shortness of breath. The patient also underwent a prostatectomy six years ago for prostatic carcinoma.

ALLERGIES: None known

CHRONIC MEDICATIONS: Ventolin and nitroglycerin as needed for chest pain

SOCIAL HISTORY: The patient is a 62-year-old male who is married and lives with his wife. He has 5 grandchildren. He is a nondrinker and a nonsmoker.

REVIEW OF SYSTEMS: The patient had normal bowels. He has had no problems with his urine since his prostatectomy. There is no hematuria or dysuria. The patient has had two colds in the past six weeks. He states that he has been having some difficulty sleeping because of the pain in his shoulder. This has limited some of the activity that he normally does, such as golf.

PHYSICAL EXAMINATION: This is a well-developed, well-nourished 62-year-old male who appears younger than his stated age.

HEENT: Aphakic, neck supple

CHEST: The lungs are clear to percussion and auscultation. The heart has normal rhythm and pulse

ABDOMEN: Abdomen reveals no masses; bowel sounds are heard

EXTREMITIES: Extremities reveal no edema

OPERATIVE REPORT—PATIENT 3

PREOPERATIVE DIAGNOSES:

1. Aphakic bullous keratopathy
2. Open-angle glaucoma
3. Chronic iritis

POSTOPERATIVE DIAGNOSES:

1. Aphakic bullous keratopathy
2. Open-angle glaucoma
3. Chronic iritis

OPERATION:

1. Aphakic penetrating keratoplasty
2. Posterior chamber intraocular lens scleral implant
3. Open-sky mechanical automated vitrectomy

ANESTHESIA: Retrobulbar block, monitored anesthesia care

COMPLICATIONS: None

INDICATIONS: This is a 62-year-old gentleman with progressive painful blurring of vision due to aphakic bullous keratopathy with glaucoma. He has undergone previous Molteno implant with poor vision and pain due to ruptured bulla. The patient is admitted for transplant vitrectomy and lens implantation of the left eye at this time. After informed consent, the patient agreed to the benefits and risks of surgery.

PROCEDURE DESCRIPTION: The patient was taken to the operating room. Under monitored anesthesia care, he was given a retrobulbar block in the standard fashion for a total of 4 cc of a 50/50 mixture 0.75% Marcaine and 4% lidocaine with Wydase.

After ensuring adequate anesthesia as well as akinesia, the patient was prepped and draped in the usual sterile ophthalmologic fashion. A wire lid speculum was inserted, and a small conjunctival peritomy was made at the two o'clock and ten o'clock hour positions to prepare for half-thickness scleral flaps for suturing a scleral-supported lens in the left eye. A Flieringa ring was then attached in the standard fashion using four interrupted 5-0 Dacron sutures. Attention was then placed to the back Mayo, and a 7.75-mm donor button was harvested, epithelial side down, in the standard fashion. Routine surveillance cultures were sent, and the donor button was placed on the Mayo stand in a Petri dish. Attention was then placed on the donor's cornea, and using a Barron-Hessburg trephine device, a 7.50-mm button was harvested under viscoelastic support. Corneoscleral scissors were used to the left and right respectively to remove the button in toto. Vitrectomy was then performed due to prolapsing vitreous, and an attempt to reposition the iris was made. However, due to loss of iris material during prior surgeries, I was unable to close the sphincter defect. After completing the vitrectomy, a scleralsupported CZ70VD 7-mm lens was secured using a 10-0 Prolene suture at the ten and two o'clock hour positions. Scleral flaps were then closed over the 10-0 Prolene to maintain a tight closure. The button was then sewn into pos ion using 16 interrupted 10-0 nylon sutures in the standard fashion. All the knots were cut short and buried in the recipient side of the host junction. A final check to make sure the chamber was watertight was unremarkable, and the Flieringa ring was removed followed by the bridle sutures. Subconjunctival Ancef and Celestone were placed, and a bandage contact lens was placed on the eye.

The patient was taken to the recovery room in good repair without complications of the above procedure.

Enter six diagnosis codes and three procedure codes.

PDX

DX2

DX3

DX4

DX5

DX6

PX1

PR2

PR3

Emergency Department E/M Mapping Scenario for Emergency Department Cases 4 and 5

Code the procedures that are done in the emergency department as well as the E/M code derived from the mapping scenario.

Point Value Key

Level 1 = 1–20
Level 2 = 21–35
Level 3 = 36–47
Level 4 = 48–60
Level 5 = > 61
Critical Care > 61 with constant physician attendance

CPT Codes

Level 1 99281 99281–25 with procedure/laboratory/radiology
Level 2 99282 99282–25 with procedure/laboratory/radiology
Level 3 99283 99283–25 with procedure/laboratory/radiology
Level 4 99284 99284–25 with procedure/laboratory/radiology
Level 5 99285 99285–25 with procedure/laboratory/radiology

Emergency Department Acuity Points

	5	10	15	20	25
Meds Given	1-2	3-5	6-7	8-9	> 10
Extent of Hx	Brief	PF	EPF	Detail	Comprehensive
Extent of Examination	Brief	PF	EPF	Detail	Comprehensive
Number of Tests Ordered	0-1	2-3	4-5	6-7	> 8
Supplies Used	1	2-3	4-5	6-7	> 8

EMERGENCY DEPARTMENT RECORD—PATIENT 4

DATE OF ADMISSION: 4/1 **DATE OF DISCHARGE:** 4/1

HISTORY (Problem Focused):

HISTORY OF PRESENT ILLNESS: This 16-year-old black female underwent piercing of her ears. The patient was removing her sweater when she accidentally pulled the earring through her ear lobe.

PAST MEDICAL HISTORY: The patient has a history of childhood asthma that has not occurred for several years.

ALLERGIES: Penicillin

CHRONIC MEDICATIONS: None

REVIEW OF SYSTEMS: The patient has been well.

PHYSICAL EXAMINATION (Problem Focused):

GENERAL APPEARANCE: This is a well-nourished 16-year-old black female in no apparent distress. HEENT normal except for 2 cm laceration of left earlobe. Neck veins flat at 40-degree angle. No nodes felt in the neck, carotids, or groin. Carotid pulsations are normal. No bruits heard in the neck. Chest clear on percussion and auscultation. Heart is not enlarged. No thrills or murmurs. Rhythm is regular. BP 130/80. Liver and spleen not palpable. No masses felt in the abdomen. No ascites noted. No edema of the extremities. Pulses in the feet are good.

IMPRESSION: Laceration of left ear lobe

PLAN: Suture laceration of ear lobe

TREATMENT: Following infiltration of the areas with Xylocaine, the laceration was closed with 2-0 Vicryl. Two suture kits were used.

DISCHARGE DIAGNOSIS: Ear lobe laceration of left ear

INSTRUCTIONS ON DISCHARGE: Demerol by mouth 50 mg every 6 hours as needed for pain. Biaxin 500 mg PO b.i.d. for 10 days. Follow-up with surgical clinic in 7 days.

Enter one diagnosis code and two procedure codes.

PDX

PP1

PR2

EMERGENCY DEPARTMENT RECORD—PATIENT 5

DATE OF ADMISSION: 6/17 **DATE OF DISCHARGE:** 6/17

HISTORY (Problem Focused):

ADMISSION HISTORY: This is a 29-year-old Asian female. She was walking down her steps when she fell. The patient complains of pain in the arm.

ALLERGIES: Penicillin

CHRONIC MEDICATIONS: Normally takes no drugs but has been taking ibuprofen every 6 hours because of painful arm.

FAMILY HISTORY: Noncontributory

SOCIAL HISTORY: The patient smokes one pack of cigarettes per day. She drinks one drink per day.

REVIEW OF SYSTEMS: The patient had hives the last time she took penicillin. Her cardiovascular, genitourinary, and gastrointestinal systems are negative.

PHYSICAL EXAMINATION (Expanded Problem Focused):

GENERAL APPEARANCE: This is an alert cooperative female in no acute distress.

HEENT: PERRLA, extraocular movements are full

NECK: Supple

CHEST: Lungs are clear. Heart has normal sinus rhythm.

ABDOMEN: Soft and nontender, no organomegaly

EXTREMITIES: Examination of the arm reveals painful movement

LABORATORY AND X-RAY DATA: Urinalysis is normal; EKG normal; chest x-ray is normal; CBC and diff show no abnormalities; x-ray of the left arm revealed a fracture of the shaft of the humerus

IMPRESSION: Fracture of the shaft of the humerus

PLAN: Reduction fracture of the humerus

TREATMENT: Following administration of conscious sedation, the patient's humeral fracture was reduced and a cast applied. One fracture tray was used.

DISCHARGE DIAGNOSIS: Fracture of the left shaft of the humerus

INSTRUCTIONS ON DISCHARGE: The patient is instructed to make an appointment with the orthopedic clinic in 3 days, to take one Percocet every 4 hours as needed for pain as per the label. Call the ER doctor if swelling or blue color of the fingers occurs. The patient is also counseled to stop smoking and was instructed to make an appointment with her primary care physician to discuss smoking cessation.

Enter two diagnosis codes and two procedure codes.

PDX ______

DX2 ______

PP1 ______

PR2 ______

AMBULATORY RECORD—PATIENT 6

Right and left heart catheterization and coronary angiography

PROCEDURE: After obtaining informed consent the patient was taken to the cardiac catheterization laboratory. The right groin was prepped and draped in the usual fashion and 2% Xylocaine was used to anesthetize. 6-French sheaths were introduced into the right femoral artery and vein and a 6-French multipurpose catheter was used for the heart catheterization, coronary angiography, and ventricular angiography. Right heart pressures and cardiac outputs were measured. A pigtail catheter was inserted into the left ventricular cavity and ventricular pressures obtained. Angiography of the right coronary artery was performed. Left ventricular angiography and aortic root angiography was performed. The patient tolerated the procedure well without complications.

DIAGNOSIS: Arteriosclerotic coronary artery disease

Enter one diagnosis code and two procedure codes.

PDX

PP1

PR2

INTERVENTIONAL RADIOLOGY REPORT—PATIENT 7

EXAMINATION: Ultrasound guided liver biopsy

HISTORY: Carcinoma of the lower right lobe of the lung

PROCEDURE: Limited real-time transabdominal ultrasound of the liver was performed. There is a 3.5 × 2.9-cm mass in the lateral segment of the left lobe of the liver. This mass is hypoechogenic with increased blood flow. Following informed consent the patient was prepped and draped in the usual manner. Using ultrasound guidance, percutaneous fine-needle aspiration biopsy of the left lobe of the liver mass was performed. The patient tolerated the procedure well.

IMPRESSION: Hypoechogenic mass in the left lobe of the liver that was successfully biopsied with ultrasound guidance

PATHOLOGY REPORT: Metastatic lung carcinoma

Enter two diagnosis codes and two procedure codes.

PDX

DX2

PP1

PR2

INPATIENT RECORD—PATIENT 8
DISCHARGE SUMMARY—PATIENT 8

DATE OF ADMISSION: 11/30 **DATE OF DISCHARGE:** 12/4

DISCHARGE DIAGNOSIS: Fractured neck of right femur

ADMISSION HISTORY: The patient is a 78-year-old male who fell on the day of admission and sustained a fracture of the neck of his right femur. The patient was admitted for a medical evaluation prior to surgical intervention.

COURSE IN HOSPITAL: Medical evaluation was obtained on admission. Patient was taken to the operating room, where an open reduction and internal fixation of the fracture of the right femur was performed. Postoperative course was unremarkable except for urinary retention, which necessitated the placement of an indwelling Foley catheter. He was discharged with the catheter in place. The patient was ambulatory, non-weight bearing with a walker at the time of discharge.

INSTRUCTIONS ON DISCHARGE: The patient is instructed to follow-up with my office in 3 days to remove staples and to begin outpatient physical therapy tomorrow. Home health services will follow this patient. Pain medications: Darvocet N 100, one tablet every 4 hours as needed for pain.

HISTORY AND PHYSICAL EXAMINATION—PATIENT 8

ADMITTED: 11/30

REASON FOR ADMISSION: Right hip pain following a fall

HISTORY OF PRESENT ILLNESS: The patient is a 78-year-old male who fell on the day of admission and sustained a fracture of the neck of his right femur. The patient was admitted for a medical evaluation prior to surgical intervention.

PAST MEDICAL HISTORY: The patient has had multiple medical problems including gastric ulcer, congestive heart failure, diverticulosis, degenerative joint disease, arteriosclerotic coronary artery disease, and mitral regurgitation.

ALLERGIES: None

CHRONIC MEDICATIONS: Lanoxin 0.125 mg, Mon. Wed., and Fri., Lasix 40 mg q. a.m., Lasix 40 mg q. p.m., Colace 200 mg q. a.m., Metamucil one teaspoon b.i.d., Zestril 10 mg every day, Zantac 150 mg PO b.i.d., nitroglycerin 0.4 mg. PRN for chest pain, Celebrex 100 mg PO b.i.d. for degenerative joint disease.

SOCIAL HISTORY: The patient is widowed with 3 children and 7 grandchildren. The patient is a nondrinker and nonsmoker.

REVIEW OF SYSTEMS: The patient has been in usual health until the day prior to admission when he fell. There has been no change in bladder and bowel functioning. Cognitively, he has experienced some confusion on and off lately.

PHYSICAL EXAMINATION: BP is 170/90, pulse 80 and regular. The patient is an elderly, thin, somewhat deaf male. His pupils are small and reactive to light. The pharynx is benign. The jugular pulse is distended but filled from above. He has no supraclavicular adenopathy. His chest is clear. On palpation the pericardium was located in his anterior axillary line with a palpable thrill. On auscultation he had a harsh grade III/VI apical systolic murmur that radiated to the apex and faintly to the lower left sternal edge. He had a soft diastolic flow murmur. His abdomen was somewhat tense without organomegaly. He had minimal peripheral edema.

CONSULTATION—PATIENT 8

DATE: 11/30

CHIEF COMPLAINT: Pain in hip

REVIEW OF SYSTEMS: The patient has been in usual health until the day prior to admission when he fell. The patient is experiencing a little more shortness of breath than usual. The patient is unsure if he felt dizzy before falling.

PHYSICAL EXAMINATION: This is an elderly, moderately nourished white male. HEENT reveals nothing abnormal. There is no adenopathy. His chest is clear with loud grade III/VI pansystolic murmur. Examination of the abdomen reveals no masses or tenderness. He had minimal peripheral edema with one leg appearing shorter than the other. Distal circulation and sensation are normal.

IMPRESSION:

History of gastric ulcer

Congestive heart failure

Diverticulosis

Degenerative joint disease

Arteriosclerotic coronary artery disease

Mitral regurgitation

PLAN: D/C NSAIDs for now in light of GI history. The patient is cleared for surgery.

PROGRESS NOTES—PATIENT 8

DATE	NOTE
11/30	Patient admitted for medical evaluation prior to ORIF. The patient is somewhat confused about the events surrounding the fall. At present he offers no other complaint. The patient currently has Bucks traction in place. If cleared for surgery, patient is scheduled for tomorrow at 1:00 P.M.
12/1	The patient is resting quietly. Medication adequate to alleviate pain in extremity.
6:30 a.m.	Operative consent signed following obtaining informed consent for surgery. All questions from patient and family answered. PREOP DX: Fracture of right femur
6:30 p.m.	POSTOP DX: Same OPERATION: Open reduction, internal fixation, fracture, right hip ANESTHESIA: Spinal and general COMPLICATIONS: None Patient sleeping. Dressings intact, hemovac in place.
8:00 p.m.	House Physician called to see patient due to inability to void. The patient appears to have postop urinary retention. Will place Foley catheter.
12/2	Events of last night noted. Will request that patient get OOB and begin physical therapy. Hemovac in place draining small amount. Patient not complaining of pain. H&H looks good. Lytes fine.
12/3	Patient has been ambulating well. Patient minimally confused due to senile dementia. Neurovascular status good. Appetite good. Dressing intact, incision healing well, no redness or inflammation.
12/4	Patient up with assistance and ambulating using walker. Incision healing well. Discharge with indwelling Foley. Home health services to assist patient following discharge. Ready for discharge today.

PHYSICIAN'S ORDERS—PATIENT 8

DATE	ORDER
11/30	Admit to floor NPO after midnight Continue present meds: Lanoxin 0.125 mg, q.d. Lasix 40 mg q. a.m. and p.m. Colace 200 mg q. a.m. Metamucil one teaspoon b.i.d. Zantac 150 mg po b.i.d. Celebrex 100 mg po b.i.d. for DJD Prep for hip surgery Medical Consult for surgical clearance 4 lb Bucks traction to continue Demerol 50 mg q. 3 to 4 hours Darvocet N 100 q. 3 to 4 hours Cross match 3 units of blood Low sodium, low-fat diet Dig level in a.m. H&H and electrolytes
12/1	Preop Meds Hold Dig this a.m. Ancef 1 g on call to OR Postop Meds Run D5W 1,000 cc q. 12 hrs Demerol 500 mg q. 3 to 4 hrs p.r.n. pain Darvocet N 100 q. 3 to 4 hours Hct and Hgb at 9:00 p.m. and in a.m. Electrolytes in a.m. Ancef 500 mg IV q. 6 hrs ×4 doses X-ray hip in a.m. Ice on hip Up in chair following x-ray Begin physical therapy tomorrow Insert Foley catheter
12/2	Consult home health services for discharge needs. Continue pain meds. Get patient OOB for ambulation with walker.
12/3	D/C IV
12/4	D/C patient. Home health services to follow.

OPERATIVE REPORT—PATIENT 8

DATE: 12/1

PREOPERATIVE DIAGNOSIS: Fracture of right femur

POSTOPERATIVE DIAGNOSIS: Same

OPERATION: Open reduction and internal fixation of fracture right hip

ANESTHESIA: Spinal and general

OPERATIVE INDICATIONS:

OPERATIVE PROCEDURE: The patient was given Ancef 1 g IV 30 minutes prior to the procedure for endocarditis/surgical prophylaxis. The patient was administered a spinal anesthesia and then placed on the fracture table in traction. X-rays revealed satisfactory position and alignment of the fracture site. The right hip was prepped with Betadine scrub and Betadine solution and draped in a sterile fashion. A straight incision was made over the lateral aspect of the right hip and carried through the subcutaneous tissue, then tensor fascia lata and vastus lateralis muscles so that the fracture could be reduced and fixation devices utilized. The lateral shaft of the femur was exposed subperiosteally. A guide wire was then placed into the neck and head of the femur and x-rays revealed a slightly inferior position. The new guide wire was obtained in satisfactory position. The lateral shaft, neck, and head of the femur were then drilled to a depth of 85 mm with the drill. An 85-mm, 140-degree and 5-degree compression nail were then inserted over which a 140-degree angle 4-hole side plate was then inserted. A compression screw was then applied after the key was inserted. The side plate was then fixed to the shaft of the femur with four screws. X-rays revealed satisfactory position and alignment of the fracture fragments and the fixation device. The wound was then well irrigated. A large hemovac drain was inserted and brought out through a separate stab wound incision. The wound was closed with a continuous #000 Vicryl suture in the vastus lateralis and tensor fascia lata layers. The subcutaneous tissue was closed with interrupted #000 Vicryl sutures and the skin was closed with staples. A compression dressing was applied. The patient tolerated the procedure well and there were no operative complications. Patient was returned to the recovery room in satisfactory condition.

LABORATORY REPORTS—PATIENT 8

HEMATOLOGY

DATE: 11/30

Specimen	Results	Normal Values
WBC	9.9	4.3-11.0
RBC	5.0	4.5-5.9
HGB	14.0	13.5-17.5
HCT	45	41-52
MCV	89	80-100
MCHC	33.9	31-57
PLT	Adequate	150-450

HEMATOLOGY

DATE: 12/1

Specimen	Results	Normal Values
WBC	7.7	4.3-11.0
RBC	4.4 L	4.5-5.9
HGB	13.2 L	13.5-17.5
HCT	41	41-52
MCV	89	80-100
MCHC	33.9	31-57
PLT	Adequate	150-450

HEMATOLOGY

DATE: 12/1

Specimen	Results	Normal Values
WBC	8.0	4.3-11.0
RBC	4.5	4.5-5.9
HGB	13.7	13.5-17.5
HCT	42	41-52
MCV	89	80-100
MCHC	33.9	31-57
PLT	Adequate	150-450

LABORATORY REPORT—PATIENT 8

CHEMISTRY

DATE: 11/30

Specimen	Results	Normal Values
GLUC	97	70–110
BUN	12	8–25
CREAT	1.0	0.5–1.5
NA	138	136–146
K	4.0	3.5–5.5
CL	109	95–110
CO_2	33 H	24–32
CA	9.1	8.4–10.5
PHOS	3.0	2.5–4.4
MG	2.0	1.6–3.0
T BILI	1.0	0.2–1.2
D BILI	0.4	0.0–0.5
PROTEIN	7.0	6.0–8.0
ALBUMIN	5.4	5.0–5.5
AST	36	0–40
ALT	44	30–65
GCT	70	15–85
LD	110	100–190
ALK PHOS	114	50–136
URIC ACID	6.0	2.2–7.7
CHOL	165	0–200
TRIG	140	10–160

LABORATORY REPORT—PATIENT 8

CHEMISTRY

DATE: 12/1

Specimen	Results	Normal Values
GLUC	97	70-110
BUN	12	8-25
CREAT	1.0	0.5-1.5
NA	134 L	136-146
K	5.6 H	3.5-5.5
CL	109	95-110
CO_2	33 H	24-32
CA	9.1	8.4-10.5
PHOS	3.0	2.5-4.4
MG	2.0	1.6-3.0
T BILI	1.0	0.2-1.2
D BILI	0.4	0.0-0.5
PROTEIN	7.0	6.0-8.0
ALBUMIN	5.4	5.0-5.5
AST	36	0-40
ALT	44	30-65
GGT	70	15-85
LD	110	100-190
ALK PHOS	114	50-136
URIC ACID	6.0	2.2-7.7
CHOL	165	0-200
TRIG	140	10-160

RADIOLOGY REPORT—PATIENT 8

DATE: 11/30

RIGHT HIP AND FEMUR: A displaced intertrochanteric fracture is noted with a mild degree of varus angulation. The adjacent skeletal structures are normal. The right femur is intact beyond the hip. There is vascular calcification.

CHEST, SUPINE: There is no gross evidence of acute inflammatory disease or congestive heart failure.

IMPRESSION: Femur and hip; slightly angulated intertrochanteric fracture; chest; no acute disease.

RADIOLOGY REPORT—PATIENT 8

DATE: 12/2

DIAGNOSIS: RIGHT HIP AND FEMUR. The displaced intertrochanteric fracture has been surgically corrected. The adjacent skeletal structures are normal.

IMPRESSION: The fracture is maintained with an orthopedic device.

Enter ten diagnosis codes and one procedure code.

PDX	
DX2	
DX3	
DX4	
DX5	
DX6	
DX7	
DX8	
DX9	
DX10	
PP1	

INPATIENT RECORD
DISCHARGE SUMMARY—PATIENT 9

DATE OF ADMISSION: 2/3 **DATE OF DISCHARGE:** 2/5

DISCHARGE DIAGNOSIS: Full-term pregnancy—delivered male infant

Patient started labor spontaneously three days before her due date. She was brought to the hospital by automobile. Labor progressed for a while but then contractions became fewer and she delivered soon after. A midline episiotomy was done. Membranes and placenta were complete. There was some bleeding but not excessive. Patient made an uneventful recovery.

HISTORY AND PHYSICAL EXAMINATION—PATIENT 9

ADMITTED: 2/3
REASON FOR ADMISSION: Full-term pregnancy
PAST MEDICAL HISTORY: Previous deliveries normal and mitral valve prolapse
ALLERGIES: None known
CHRONIC MEDICATIONS: None
FAMILY HISTORY: Heart disease—father
SOCIAL HISTORY: The patient is married and has one other child living with her.
REVIEW OF SYSTEMS:
- **SKIN:** Normal
- **HEAD-SCALP:** Normal
- **EYES:** Normal
- **ENT:** Normal
- **NECK:** Normal
- **BREASTS:** Normal
- **THORAX:** Normal
- **LUNGS:** Normal
- **HEART:** Slight midsystolic click with late systolic murmur II/VI
- **ABDOMEN:** Normal

IMPRESSION: Good health with term pregnancy. History of mitral valve prolapse—asymptomatic.

PROGRESS NOTES—PATIENT 9

DATE	NOTE
2/3	Admit to Labor and Delivery. MVP stable. Patient progressing well. Delivered at 1:15 p.m. one full-term male infant.
2/4	Patient doing well. MVP prolapse stable. The perineum is clean and dry, incision intact.
2/5	Will discharge to home

PHYSICIAN'S ORDERS—PATIENT 9

DATE	ORDER
2/3	Admit to Labor and Delivery
	1,000 cc 5% D/LR
	May ambulate
	Type and screen
	CBC
	May have ice chips
2/5	Discharge patient to home.

DELIVERY RECORD—PATIENT 9

DATE: 2/3

The patient was 3 cm dilated when admitted. The duration of the first stage of labor was 6 hours, second stage was 14 minutes, third stage was 5 minutes. She was given local anesthesia. An episiotomy was performed with repair. There were no lacerations. The cord was wrapped once around the baby's neck, but did not cause compression. The mother and liveborn baby were discharged from the delivery room in good condition.

LABORATORY REPORT—PATIENT 9

HEMATOLOGY

DATE: 2/3

Specimen	Results	Normal Values
WBC	5.2	4.3-11.0
RBC	4.9	4.5-5.9
HGB	13.8	13.5-17.5
HCT	45	41-52
MCV	93	80-100
MCHC	41	31-57
PLT	255	150-450

Enter four diagnosis codes and one procedure code.

PDX

DX2

DX3

DX4

PP1

INPATIENT RECORD
DISCHARGE SUMMARY—PATIENT 10

DATE OF ADMISSION: 1/31 **DATE OF DISCHARGE:** 2/3

DISCHARGE DIAGNOSIS: Right lower lobe pneumonia due to gram-negative bacteria, resistant to erythromycin

ADMISSION HISTORY: This is a 56-year-old insulin-requiring diabetic female whose diabetes is out of control whom we have been following for hypertension, degenerative joint disease, aortic stenosis and diabetic retinopathy. Over the past three days she has noted increased cough and chest congestion with a fever of approximately 102 degrees. She was found to have a right lower lobe infiltrate and was started on therapy with erythromycin. Despite initial therapy, the patient's clinical status has worsened over the past 24 hours.

COURSE IN HOSPITAL: Patient was admitted with the diagnosis of right lower lobe pneumonia. She was begun on intravenous ceftriaxone. Because of difficulties with venous access, patient was switched to intramuscular ceftriaxone on her third hospital day.

By 2/3 the patient was afebrile and her cough had diminished. Her blood pressure was well controlled at 140/74.

INSTRUCTIONS ON DISCHARGE: Follow-up with me by phone in three days and in my office in two weeks. Repeat chest x-ray to be done then.

MEDICATIONS:

1. Calan SR 180 mg b.i.d.
2. Zestril 20 mg PO q. a.m.
3. NPH Insulin, 30 units, sub q., a.m.
4. Levoquin 500 mg PO daily ×10 days
5. Celebrex 100 mg PO b.i.d.

HISTORY AND PHYSICAL EXAMINATION—PATIENT 10

ADMITTED: 1/31

REASON FOR ADMISSION: Physical examination on admission revealed a well-developed, acutely ill appearing black female.

HISTORY OF PRESENT ILLNESS: A 56-year-old diabetic followed for hypertension and diabetic retinopathy. Over the past three days she has noted increased cough and chest congestion with a fever of approximately 102 degrees. She was found to have a right lower lobe infiltrate and was begun on therapy with erythromycin. Despite initial therapy, the patient's clinical status worsened over the past 24 hours and hospitalization was recommended.

PAST MEDICAL HISTORY: Hypertension, degenerative joint disease in both knees, and moderate aortic stenosis.

ALLERGIES: Dust

CHRONIC MEDICATIONS: CalanSR 180 mg po b.i.d., Insulin (NPH), Zestril 20 mg PO daily, Celebrex 100 mg PO b.i.d.

FAMILY HISTORY: Notable for hypertension in mother

SOCIAL HISTORY: Noncontributory

PHYSICAL EXAMINATION:

GENERAL APPEARANCE: The patient is a well-developed black female in moderate distress.

VITAL SIGNS: T 102, P 80, R 16, BP 150/80

SKIN: Warm and dry

HEENT: Significant for mildly inflamed mucous membranes. Retinopathy evident in both eyes.

NECK: Supple. Symmetrical with no bruits

LUNGS: Coarse rhonchi bilaterally, right greater than left

HEART: Regular rate and rhythm, positive S1, positive III/VI SEM

ABDOMEN: Soft, nontender, no mass

GENITALIA: Deferred

RECTAL: Deferred

EXTREMITIES: No edema

NEUROLOGIC: Normal

HISTORY AND PHYSICAL EXAMINATION—PATIENT 10

LABORATORY DATA:

1. EKG: NSR, widespread ST-T wave abnormalities, LV hypertrophy
2. CBC: Hgb 13, Hct 38, WBC 12.8
3. Glucose: 281
4. Urinalysis: Unremarkable
5. Sputum: Gram stain—a few WBCs, moderate gram-negative rods

IMPRESSION:

1. Right lower lobe pneumonia possibly due to gram-negative bacteria
2. Diabetes mellitus on insulin—uncontrolled
3. Hypertension—atable
4. Degenerative joint disease—atable
5. Moderate aortic stenosis

PLAN: Admit, IV antibiotics for pneumonia. Monitor blood sugars.

PROGRESS NOTES—PATIENT 10

DATE	NOTE
1/31	Patient admitted for cough associated with increased temperature with chest x-ray indicative of pneumonia. Will obtain sputum culture and begin on ceftriaxone. Will monitor blood pressure and blood sugars. Will use sliding scale to bring blood sugar into control. Patient with recent echocardiogram as outpatient that showed stable aortic stenosis.
2/1	The patient is responding well. Will request diabetic education nurse to meet with her and set up an appointment for classes following this admission.
2/2	Sputum culture reveals gram-negative bacteria as suspected. Patient's temperature is down. Patient resting comfortably. Blood sugar better.
2/3	Blood sugar with increasing control today. The importance of appropriate diet emphasized. Will discharge with p.o. antibiotics.

PHYSICIAN'S ORDERS—PATIENT 10

DATE	ORDER
1/31/20XX	Admit to 3 South DX: Pneumonia Please give ceftriaxone 1 g q 8 hours IV ADA diet CBC and SMA CalanSR 50 mg in a.m. with orange juice Zestril 2 in a.m. Celebrex 100 mg po BID Accucheck before meals and before bedtime Chest x-ray Sliding scale for insulin as follows: Below 120 give 4 units of regular 120–200 give 6 units of regular insulin 200–300 give 8 units of regular insulin Above 300, call physician
2/1/20XX	Change insulin to 40 NPH units sq in a.m. today. Consult diabetic nurse to see patient and set up classes following admission.
2/2/20XX	Continue insulin to 40 NPH units sq in a.m. today.
2/2/20XX	D/C IV and switch to ceftriaxone 1 g IM q. 24 hrs
2/3/20XX	Discharge to home.

LABORATORY REPORTS—PATIENT 10
MICROBIOLOGY

DATE	TEST TYPE	
1/31/20XX	**SOURCE:**	
	SITE:	
	GRAM STAIN RESULTS: Sputum	
	CULTURE RESULTS: Slight WBC's, Slight Epi's	
	Many gram-negative rods	
	sl. gram-negative diplococci	
	sl. gram-positive cocci in clusters	
	SUSCEPTIBILITY:	S
	AMPICILLIN	S
	CEFAZOLIN	S
	CEFOTAXIME	S
	CEFTRIAXONE	S
	CEFUROXIME	S
	CEPHALOTHIN	S
	CIPROFLOXACIN	S
	ERYTHROMYCIN	R
	GENTAMICIN	S
	OXACILLIN	S
	PENICILLIN	S
	PIPERACILLIN	S
	TETRACYCLINE	S
	TOBRAMYCIN	S
	TRIMETH/SULF	S
	VANCOMYCIN	S

S = SUSCEPTIBLE
R = RESISTANT
I = INTERMEDIATE
M = MODERATELY SUSCEP

RADIOLOGY REPORT—PATIENT 10

DATE: 1/31/20XX

HISTORY DIAGNOSIS: Pneumonia

FINDINGS: There is slight overexpansion of the lungs. The pulmonary vasculature is normal. The heart is not enlarged. There is lower lobe infiltrate in the right lung.

IMPRESSION: Right lower lobe pneumonia

EKG REPORT—PATIENT 10

DATE: 1/31/20XX

DIAGNOSIS: Pneumonia

INTERPRETATION: EKG: NSR, widespread ST-T wave abnormalities, LV hypertrophy

LABORATORY REPORT—PATIENT 10

CHEMISTRY

DATE: 1/31/20XX

Specimen	Results	Normal Values
GLUC	281 H	70–110
CREAT	0.67	0.5–1.5
NA	142	136–146
K	4.8	3.5–5.5
CL	108	95–110
CO_2	29	24–32
CA	9.5	8.4–10.5
PHOS	3.8	2.5–4.4
MG	2.8	1.6–3.0
T BILI	1.0	0.2–1.2
D BILI	0.3	0.0–0.5
PROTEIN	6.5	6.0–8.0
ALBUMIN	5.1	5.0–5.5
AST	38	0–40
ALT	54	30–65
GGT	50	15–85
LD	180	100–190
ALK PHOS	102	50–136
URIC ACID	4.5	2.2–7.7
CHOL	89	0–200
TRIG	101	10–160

LABORATORY REPORT—PATIENT 10
URINALYSIS

DATE: 1/31

Test	Result	Ref Range
SP GRAVITY	1.007	1.005-1.035
PH	7.0	5-7
PROT	NEG	NEG
GLUC	NEG	NEG
KETONES	NEG	NEG
BILI	NEG	NEG
BLOOD	NEG	NEG
LEU EST	NEG	NEG
NITRATES	NEG	NEG
RED SUBS	NEG	NEG

LABORATORY REPORTS—PATIENT 10
HEMATOLOGY

DATE: 1/31

Specimen	Results	Normal Values
WBC	12.8 H	4.3-11.0
RBC	5.5	4.5-5.9
HGB	13.0 L	13.5-17.5
HCT	38 L	41-52
MCV	90	80-100
MCHC	41	31-57
PLT	251	150-450

BLOOD GLUCOSE MONITORING RECORD—PATIENT 10		
1/31/20XX	11:00 a.m.	310
	4:00 p.m.	300
	9:00 p.m.	290
2/1/20XX	7:00 a.m.	150
	11:00 a.m.	175
	4:00 p.m.	145
	9:00 p.m.	175
2/2/20XX	7:00 a.m.	140
	11:00 a.m.	135
	4:00 p.m.	160
	9:00 p.m.	150
2/3/20XX	7:00 a.m.	135
	11:00 a.m.	150
	4:00 p.m.	130

Enter eight diagnosis codes.

PDX

DX2

DX3

DX4

DX5

DX6

DX7

DX8

INPATIENT RECORD
DISCHARGE SUMMARY—PATIENT 11

DATE OF ADMISSION: 2/3 **DATE OF DISCHARGE:** 2/4

DISCHARGE DIAGNOSIS: Malignant ascites from metastatic adenocarcinoma of the colon

COURSE IN HOSPITAL: This 59-year-old white female patient was admitted for continuous infusion chemotherapy with 5-FU and Leucovoran. This was done under the care of Dr. ZXY. The patient tolerated her chemotherapy very well. She had no complications throughout her hospital course, and she was discharged to be followed further as an outpatient by her oncologist.

INSTRUCTIONS ON DISCHARGE: Follow up in the office.

HISTORY AND PHYSICAL EXAMINATION—PATIENT 11

ADMITTED: 2/3/20XX
REASON FOR ADMISSION: Chemotherapy
HISTORY OF PRESENT ILLNESS: The patient is a 59-year-old white female with carcinomatosis and malignant ascites from colon carcinoma. She is admitted for continuous chemotherapy. The patient has a sigmoid colostomy and has had multiple abdominal surgeries for carcinoma, the first one was an anterior and posterior repair in 1982. She had 6 weeks of radiation therapy completed two years ago and has been on weekly chemotherapy consisting of 5-FU and methotrexate recently. Because of increasing abdominal girth, she was admitted in June 1987, and diagnosed with malignant ascites and carcinomatosis. At that time, she had an extensive evaluation including an upper gastrointestinal series, barium enema, CT scan, and ultrasound of the abdomen. She was told she had adhesions causing a partial obstruction. No further surgery was pursued. For the past week, she has complained of frequent vomiting. Her weight has decreased another 6 pounds. She denies any abdominal pain. She has occasional diarrhea for which she takes Questran. She has had no blood in her colostomy drainage.
PAST MEDICAL HISTORY: No hypertension, myocardial infarction, diabetes, or peptic ulcer disease. Anterior and posterior repair in 1982, colectomy, cholecystectomy, appendectomy, hysterectomy with bilateral salpingo-oophorectomy for uterine fibroids in 1968.
ALLERGIES: None
CHRONIC MEDICATIONS: Pancrease three times a day; Questran as needed for diarrhea; Os-Cal 2 × per day, 250 mg
FAMILY HISTORY: Mother died at age 80. Father died of colon cancer at age 60.
SOCIAL HISTORY: Prior to that time, she smoked a pack a day for 20 years. She denies any alcohol intake. She works in the shipping department.
REVIEW OF SYSTEMS: Unremarkable
PHYSICAL EXAMINATION: An alert, white female in no acute distress
GENERAL APPEARANCE:

SKIN, HEAD, EYES, EARS, NOSE, THROAT: Pupils are equal, reactive to light and accommodation. Extraocular movements are intact. Fundi are benign. Tympanic membranes are normal.
MOUTH: No oral lesions are seen.
HEENT: Within normal limits.
NECK: Carotids are plus 2 with no bruits. Thyroid is normal. There is no adenopathy at present.
LUNGS: Clear
HEART: Regular sinus rhythm. No murmur, rub, or gallop.
BREASTS: A small, approximately 3 mm, cystic lesion the medial aspect of her left breast at around eight o'clock. It is freely movable and nontender. There are no axillary nodes.
ABDOMEN: Distended. Sigmoid colostomy present. Right lower quadrant induration is present. There is no abdominal tenderness. There is no hepatosplenomegaly. Bowel sounds are normal.
PULSES: Femorals are plus 2 with no bruits. There are good pedal pulses bilaterally.
GENITALIA: Normal
RECTAL: Deferred
EXTREMITIES: No edema
NEUROLOGIC: Deep tendon reflexes are plus 2 throughout

LABORATORY DATA: Pending
IMPRESSION:
Abdominal carcinomatosis retro-peritoneum and peritoneum from colon cancer
Small left breast cyst
PLAN: The patient will be admitted for continuous chemotherapy.

PROGRESS NOTES—PATIENT 11

DATE	NOTE
2/3	Patient tolerating chemo well. No complaints offered.
2/4	Patient well hydrated, nausea and vomiting under control. Will discharge.

PHYSICIAN'S ORDERS—PATIENT 11

DATE	ORDER
2/3	Chemotherapy protocol in D5W
	Compazine 5 mg now, then Q4H prn
2/4	Discontinue IV
	Discharge the patient.

Enter nine diagnosis codes and one procedure code.

PDX

DX2

DX3

DX4

DX5

DX6

DX7

DX8

DX9

PP1

INPATIENT RECORD
DISCHARGE SUMMARY—PATIENT 12

DATE OF ADMISSION: 1/3 **DATE OF DISCHARGE:** 1/7

DISCHARGE DIAGNOSIS: Recurrent carcinoma, left lung

This is a 63-year-old female who is two years status post left upper lobe resection for adenocarcinoma. Pathology at that time revealed a positive bronchial margin of resection. She was treated with postop radiation and has done extremely well. She has remained asymptomatic with no postoperative difficulty. Follow up serial CT scans have revealed a new lesion in the apical portion of the left lung, which on needle biopsy was positive for adenocarcinoma. She was admitted specifically for a left thoracotomy and possible pneumonectomy.

PAST MEDICAL HISTORY: Positive for tobacco abuse 2 PPD × 30 years in the past. Significant for a right parotidectomy and also significant for hypertension, degenerative joint disease of lumbar spine, and chronic pulmonary disease. The patient also suffered a stroke in the left brain with resulting hemiparesis three years ago. Medications on discharge: Tenormin 25 mg once a day, Calan SR 240 mg twice a day, Moduretic one tablet q. day and K-Dur 10 meq q. day, Proventil MDI 2 puffs PO q.i.d. p.r.n., Azacort MDI 2 puffs PO t.i.d., Vioxx 25 mg PO daily.

PHYSICAL EXAMINATION: Revealed a well-healed right parotid incision. No supraclavicular adenopathy. She has a healed left posterior lateral thoracotomy scar. Impression is that of local recurrence, status post left upper lobectomy. She is to undergo a left pneumonectomy.

OPERATIVE FINDINGS AND HOSPITAL COURSE: There was a large mass in the remaining lung, extensive mediastinal fibrosis, bronchial margin free by frozen section. Following surgery she was placed in the intensive care unit postoperatively. The chest tube was removed on postoperative day number two.

She experienced some EKG changes consistent with acute nontransmural MI. Cardiology was consulted, and she was started on nitroglycerin and IV heparin. She was eventually weaned from her oxygen therapy.

She was started on regular diet and was discharged in good condition. Her wound was clean and dry.

INSTRUCTIONS ON DISCHARGE: Discharged home with instructions to follow up with cardiology next week. Also follow up with me in the office.

HISTORY AND PHYSICAL EXAMINATION—PATIENT 12

Admitted: 1/3

HISTORY OF PRESENT ILLNESS: Patient is a 63-year-old right-handed female with history of recurrent adenocarcinoma of apical segment of left upper lobe of lung. She has received radiation therapy to her chest. She weighs 123 pounds. She also has chronic obstructive pulmonary disease.

REVIEW OF SYSTEMS: She can climb two flights of steps with minimal difficulties. She has a significant underbite. She has stiffness in lower spine, worse in the a.m. She has hypertension and took her Tenormin 25 mg, Calan SR 240 mg this a.m.

PAST SURGICAL HISTORY: She had a right parotidectomy seven years ago and was told they needed to use a "very small" ETT. Two years ago she underwent a left upper lobe resection at this facility. Previous medical records are being requested.

ALLERGIES: She is allergic to sulfa. Postoperatively last time she received Demerol. She also had hallucinations in the ICU for several days. She blames the hallucinations on the Demerol. The only allergy sign was hallucinations.

PHYSICAL EXAMINATION: Revealed a well-healed right parotid incision. No supraclavicular adenopathy. She has a healed left posterior lateral thoracotomy scar. Impression is that of local recurrence, status post left upper lobectomy. She is to undergo a left completion pneumonectomy, muscle flap coverage of bronchial stump. The patient has hemiparesis in the right extremities.

IMPRESSION: Recurrent carcinoma left lower lobe of lung

PLAN: Pneumonectomy of left lung. The patient is agreeable to general endotracheal anesthesia or the use of epidural narcotic. She is agreeable to postoperative ventilation if necessary.

PROGRESS NOTES—PATIENT 12	
DATE	**NOTE**
1/3	Attending Physician: Admit for recurrent lung carcinoma, s/p radiation therapy. Consent signed for pneumonectomy. Epidural morphine usage postop explained to and discussed with the patient. She is agreeable. Anesthesia Preop: Patient evaluated and examined. General anesthesia chosen. Patient agrees. Will provide postop epidural morphine for pain management s/p thoracotomy. Attending Physician: Procedure Note: Preop Dx: Local recurrence of carcinoma of the lung Postop Dx: Same Procedure: Pneumonectomy with muscle flap coverage of bronchial stump Complications: R/O Intraop MI Anesthesia Postop: Patient in stable condition following GEA with possible intraoperative MI due to hypotension. CPK to be evaluated as available. Patient comfortable with epidural morphine. No adverse effects of anesthesia experienced.
1/4	Attending Physician: Path report confirms recurrent adenocarcinoma. Patient stable but with persistent hypotension resolving slowly—will consult cardiology. CPK MB positive. Incision clean and dry. COPD stable, arthritis stable. Cardiology Consult: The patient has resolving intraoperative myocardial infarction. Will continue to monitor.
1/5	Attending Physician: Looks and feels well, weaning off morphine. Blood pressure stable. Left pleural space expanding and filling space. Chest tube removed, epidural cath removed. Cardiology Consult: The patient looking and feeling better.
1/6	Attending Physician: Patient stable for discharge in a.m. Cardiology to follow.

OPERATIVE REPORT—PATIENT 12

DATE: 1/3

OPERATION: Pneumonectomy

PREOPERATIVE DIAGNOSIS: Recurrent carcinoma of left lung

POSTOPERATIVE DIAGNOSIS: Same

ANESTHESIA: General endotracheal anesthesia

OPERATIVE FINDINGS: There was a large mass in the left lower lobe.

The patient was prepped and draped in the usual fashion. Following thoracotomy the left lung was completely removed. A muscle flap coverage was used for the bronchial stump. During the procedure the patient experienced an episode of hypotension, watch for resulting MI. The patient was fluid resuscitated and sent to the recovery room in good condition.

PATHOLOGY REPORT—PATIENT 12

DATE: 1/3

SPECIMEN: Left lung, resected

CLINICAL DATA: This is a 63-year-old female with recurrent disease on CT scan.

DIAGNOSIS: Adenocarcinoma of the apical portion of the lung, bronchial margin is free of disease.

PHYSICIAN'S ORDERS—PATIENT 12

DATE	ORDER
1/3	Admit to surgical floor
	Standard orders for thoracotomy
	Tenormin 25 mg q.d.
	Calan SR 240 mg twice a day
	Moduretic one tab. q.d.
	K-Dur 10 meq q.d. in a.m.
	Vioxx 25 mg PO daily in a.m.
	Proventil (albuterol) MDI 2 puffs PO q.i.d.
	Azmacort MDI 2 puffs PO q.i.d.
	CBC
	Postop Orders:
	Admit to ICU
	Serial CPK stat
	CBC
	SMA 12
	Anesthesia:
	Morphine pump ad lib
	D5NSS 100 cc/hr
	Strict input and output documentation
1/4	Attending MD: Consult Cardiology
	Cardiology: Lasix 20 mg b.i.d. PO
	D/C IV
1/5	Transfer to floor
	Continue meds
1/6	Discharge patient in a.m.

LABORATORY REPORTS—PATIENT 12

HEMATOLOGY

DATE: 1/3

Specimen	Results	Normal Values
WBC	5.7	4.3-11.0
RBC	5.0	4.5-5.9
HGB	15.6	13.5-17.5
HCT	47	41-52
MCV	89	80-100
MCHC	42	31-57
PLT	300	150-450

HEMATOLOGY

DATE: 1/4

Specimen	Results	Normal Values
WBC	5.6	4.3-11.0
RBC	4.0 L	4.5-5.9
HGB	13.4 L	13.5-17.5
HCT	40 L	41-52
MCV	82	80-100
MCHC	33	31-57
PLT	200	150-450

LABORATORY REPORT—PATIENT 12

CHEMISTRY

DATE: 1/3

Specimen	Results	Normal Values
GLUC	90	70–110
BUN	27 H	8–25
CREAT	1.0	0.5–1.5
NA	138	136–146
K	4.0	3.5–5.5
CL	100	95–110
CO_2	28	24–32
CA	8.9	8.4–10.5
PHOS	2.9	2.5–4.4
MG	2.0	1.6–3.0
T BILI	1.0	0.2–1.2
D BILI	0.04	0.0–0.5
PROTEIN	7.0	6.0–8.0
ALBUMIN	5.3	5.0–5.5
AST	35	0–40
ALT	50	30–65
MB	7 H, 15 H, 12 H, 9 H	0–5.0
CPK	221, 250 H, 275 H, 230	21–232

RADIOLOGY REPORT—PATIENT 12

DATE: 1/3

Chest x-ray: Reveals mass in the left lower lobe. There are surgical clips in the thorax from apparent previous surgery. The thoracic organs are midline and the vasculature is normal.

IMPRESSION: Carcinoma LLL, no congestive heart failure.

RADIOLOGY REPORT—PATIENT 12

DATE: 1/4

Chest x-ray: Reveals absence of left lung. Other architecture is normal other than postoperative changes. The thoracic organs are midline and the vasculature is normal.

IMPRESSION: Postop changes consistent with lobectomy; no congestive heart failure.

EKG REPORT—PATIENT 12
DATE: 1/3
Normal sinus rhythm
DATE: 1/4
There are nonspecific ST changes consistent with possible evolving myocardial infarction.
DATE: 1/5
Possible acute myocardial infarction, please correlate with other clinical findings.

Enter ten diagnosis codes and one procedure code.

PDX	
DX2	
DX3	
DX4	
DX5	
DX6	
DX7	
DX8	
DX9	
DX10	
PP1	

INPATIENT RECORD
DISCHARGE SUMMARY—PATIENT 13

DATE OF ADMISSION: 4/19 **DATE OF DISCHARGE:** 4/24

DISCHARGE DIAGNOSIS:

Acute myocardial infarction

Hyperlipidemia

Complete heart block

Upper gastrointestinal hemorrhage

Arteriosclerotic heart disease

ADMISSION HISTORY: This is a 45-year-old white male with a history of hyperlipidemia and tobacco use. He presented to the hospital with an acute myocardial infarction. He was treated with intravenous TPA and had a reperfusion. The patient continued to have chest pain with an inferior ST elevation on EKG.

COURSE IN HOSPITAL: The patient sustained an acute myocardial infarction. The patient presented with an acute myocardial infarction and underwent catheterization. The patient was found to have stenosis of the mid right coronary artery and right distal coronary artery. The left coronary branches have minimal noncritical disease. The left ventricular ejection fraction was approximately 45% with inferior wall hypokinesis.

The patient had a successful stent PTCA to the mid-RCA with a stent. I initially attempted to dilate with a balloon, but the results were inadequate and proceeded to place a 4.0-mm J&J stent. The patient continued to have anginal symptomatology and for this reason was taken to the OR for CABG ×2. He did well after the CABG ×2 without any anginal symptoms.

The patient also had gastrointestinal bleeding following the PTCA. The patient developed retching and hematemesis and anemia for which he required blood transfusion. The probable cause of the nausea and vomiting was a reaction to anesthesia. Upper endoscopy revealed no evidence of peptic ulcer disease.

At the present time the patient has been treated with aspirin and Ticlid and has been doing very well. The plan is to discharge him home with follow up in my office next week.

INSTRUCTIONS ON DISCHARGE: Follow up in 1 week in my office. Medications include; aspirin 1 tablet per day, Ticlid 250 mg twice per day, Tagamet 400 mg twice per day and sublingual nitroglycerin as needed for chest pain. Condition upon discharge is stable. Activity is restricted until cardiac rehabilitation.

HISTORY AND PHYSICAL EXAMINATION—PATIENT 13

ADMITTED: 4/19
Acute myocardial infarction
Complete heart block
Ventricular ectopy
Possible ASHD

REASON FOR ADMISSION: Pain in chest

HISTORY OF PRESENT ILLNESS: This is a pleasant 45-year-old male with a history of hyperlipidemia and previous tobacco use. He also has a family history of coronary artery disease. He denies any prior history of coronary artery disease, myocardial infarction, or CVAs. The patient has been essentially very healthy, except for occasional skipped heartbeat in the past for which he has never taken any medications. The patient is presently on no medications.

Two days ago, he started complaining of a dull chest ache that appeared to radiate to his left arm and lasted for a few minutes. He was brought to the emergency department and was noted to have an acute inferior myocardial infarction with complete heart block. I was consulted to evaluate the patient and proceeded with administration of TPA therapy and IV Atropine for complete heart block. At the present time the patient is in sinus rhythm and is presently receiving IV TPA. He denies any melena, hematochezia. Denies any shortness of breath, PND, orthopnea.

PAST MEDICAL HISTORY: He denies any history of hypertension or diabetes. He has a history of high cholesterol. He states that he had his cholesterol checked approximately 3 months ago and it was around 310. He used to smoke tobacco, one pack a day for 20 years. He quit smoking 6 months ago. He denies any history of coronary artery disease, myocardial infarction, or cerebrovascular accident.

He has a history of heart palpitations that he describes as skipped heartbeat in the past for which he is not taking any medications. He has never had an evaluation.

He has a history of kidney stones 2 years ago. He denies any history of peptic ulcer disease. He has a history of hemorrhoidal bleeding in the past. The last episode of bleeding was 6 or 7 months ago.

The patient denies any trauma or recent surgery.

ALLERGIES: Patient has no known drug allergies.

CHRONIC MEDICATIONS: None

SOCIAL HISTORY: He quit tobacco 6 months ago and denies alcohol abuse. He is a construction worker.

REVIEW OF SYSTEMS: Denies melena, hematochezia, hematemesis and he denies change in weight.

PHYSICAL EXAMINATION: This is a pleasant gentleman who appears slightly diaphoretic and is expressing having mild chest pain which is better from admission. He is presently receiving IV TPA. Vital signs are as follows: Blood pressure is 100/70; heart rate in the 80s. The neck shows no JVD, no carotid bruits. The lungs are clear and heart is regular rate with S4 gallop rhythm and no murmurs. The abdomen is soft and nontender. Extremities show no edema. The pulses of his femoral and dorsalis pedis are 2+ bilaterally. Neurological examination reveals an alert and oriented male ×3.

LABORATORY DATA: SMA-7, sodium 138, potassium 3.7, BUN 7, creatinine 0.9. CBC showed a white blood cell count of 12. Hematocrit 37, hemoglobin 13. Platelet count is 312. His EKG showed complete heart block with significant ST elevation in the inferior leads with reciprocal changes in the anteroseptal leads, consistent with an acute inferior wall myocardial infarction. His chest x-ray is pending.

IMPRESSION AND PLAN: Acute myocardial infarction that appears to have started around 10:30 in the morning. He presented very early to the emergency department and was treated aggressively with intravenous TPA, intravenous aspirin, intravenous nitroglycerin.

We will continue the TPA and begin lidocaine. We will obtain cardiac enzymes and admit to CCU. The patient will need cardiac catheterization evaluated within 48 hours. If symptoms recur or patient does not have evidence of reperfusion will need urgent cardiac catheterization. If heart block occurs, will treat with intravenous Atropine on a p.r.n. basis. We will check a cholesterol and lipid profile in the hospital.

CONSULTATION—PATIENT 13

DATE: 4/20

CHIEF COMPLAINT: Vomiting blood

REVIEW OF SYSTEMS: This 45-year-old white male was seen in consultation because of GI bleeding. The patient was admitted one day ago with acute myocardial infarction. He was treated with TPA and later went to cardiac catheterization where he was found to have a lesion of the mid RCA and distal RCA. Today the patient exhibited hematemesis with retching. He has no past history of ulcer disease or GI bleeding.

PHYSICAL EXAMINATION: Physical examination reveals an adult male lying in bed. Blood pressure is 120/80, pulses 60. HEENT: Pale. LUNGS: Clear. HEART: Regular rate and rhythm. ABDOMEN: Benign.

LABORATORY: WBC is 12, hemoglobin 12, and hematocrit 37

IMPRESSION: Upper GI bleeding; rule out ulcer disease

RECOMMENDATION: We will perform an upper endoscopy to be performed today after informed consent is obtained. Further recommendations are to follow.

PROGRESS NOTES—PATIENT 13

DATE	NOTE
4/19	This is a 45-year-old white male with a history of increased cholesterol, no prior coronary artery disease, MI or CVA. He presented with acute ischemia and heart block. He was given IV TPA; 1–1½ hours after TPA he had severe chest pain with elevated ST inferior leads. He was treated emergently for urgent catheter and PTCA. Post catheter/stent Procedure: Left heart catheter, coronary angio, left ventricular angiography Results: Normal LCA, 99% mid-RCA and 70 stenosis distal RCA, successful stent PTCA to mid RCA with excellent results.
4/20	Cardiac: Patient continues to have pain. Will prepare for CABG when patient stable from GI perspective. GI: The patient experienced vomiting with flecks of blood after the cardiac catheterization. In light of apparent acute blood loss anemia will check for peptic ulcer. Probable reaction to anesthetics. Endoscopy Note: Preop: Gastrointestinal bleeding Postop: Gastrointestinal bleeding, etiology unknown Procedure: EGD Complications: None
4/21	Patient is scheduled for the OR today. Bleeding stable. OP Note: Preop: Critical stenosis of the mid-RCA and distal RCA Postop: Same Operation: CABG ×2 Complications: None
4/22	Patient recovering well. No chest pain or shortness of breath. The wound looks good. Will monitor blood loss anemia. The patient declines blood transfusion.
4/23	Chest clear, no chest pain, abdomen is soft with bowel sounds. Will transfer to the floor.
4/24	Wound healing well, patient OOB ambulating, no chest pain, lungs clear.
4/25	Will discharge today. Patient to follow up in 1 week.

PHYSICIAN'S ORDERS—PATIENT 13

DATE	ORDER
4/19	Admit to CCU
	DX: Acute MI
	Cardiac enzymes q. 8 hours ×3
	CBC q. day ×3
	Meds:
	IV nitro @ 20 ug/min
	ASA 325 mg PO q. day
	Ticlid 250 mg PO b.i.d.
	Xanax 0.25 mg PO t.i.d. p.r.n.
	Restoril 30 mgs PO q. h p.r.n. for sleep
	Zantac 150 mg PO b.i.d.
	Daily PT and INR, PTT
	Diet: cardiac
	Vital signs q. 15 min ×8 then q.i.d.
	Bed rest
	02 at 2 L/min.
	NS at 150 cc/hr for 10 hours
4/20	Lopressor 25 mg PO t.i.d.
	Social worker consult re: payment issues
	CBC at 6 p.m.
	NPO for now
	Possible endoscopy
	Postendoscopy orders
	Watch VS
	Resume previous orders
	No heparin or TPA
	Hgb and Hct q. 6 h
	NS at 125 cc/hr
	D/C ASA, Ticlid for now
	Tagamet drip per protocol
4/21	Postop CABG orders:
	Continue present ventilator settings
	Daily electrolytes and CBC
	Morphine sulfate 15 mg PO q. 4h p.r.n.
	TED stockings
	Weigh patient daily
	Routine weaning in a.m.
	Lidocaine 3 g/min
	Continue Tagamet drip

PHYSICIAN'S ORDERS—PATIENT 13 (continued)

4/22	Decrease Lidocaine to 2 g/min Extubate patient as soon as weaned from ventilator Chest tubes to low suction Oxygen face mask 4 L/min Encourage incentive spirometry
4/23	Nutrition consult re: low-fat, low-salt diet D/C Tagamet drip to 250 mg q. 6 Benadryl p.r.n. for sleep Consult cardiac rehab
4/24	D/C oxygen Consult home healthcare for postsurgical monitoring
4/25	Discharge patient

OPERATIVE REPORT—PATIENT 13

DATE: 4/21

PREOPERATIVE DIAGNOSIS: Critical stenosis of mid right coronary artery and distal right coronary artery

POSTOPERATIVE DIAGNOSIS: Same

OPERATION: Coronary bypass ×2 using saphenous vein from aorta to right mid coronary artery and distal right coronary artery

ANESTHESIA: General

Under general anesthesia with arterial and pulmonary artery monitoring with sterile prep and drape, a sterile midline sternotomy was performed. The pericardium was opened. Purse-string sutures were placed in the ascending aorta and the right atrium. Extracorporeal circulation was undertaken at this point. The saphenous vein was harvested from the right leg in the usual fashion. The patient was then placed on cardiopulmonary bypass. Cardioplegia was affected. The right coronary artery was dissected. Using a 6-0 Prolene suture an end-to-side anastomosis was created between the right mid coronary artery and the aorta. A second opening for end to side anastomosis was performed from the aorta to the distal right coronary artery. Following spontaneous contraction of the heart the patient was removed from cardiopulmonary bypass. Approximating the pericardium then began closure. Hemostasis was obtained. The sternum was approximated with a parasternal wire and fascia and skin with vicryl. The patient tolerated the procedure well and was transferred to the recovery room in stable condition.

ENDOSCOPY REPORT—PATIENT 13

DATE: 4/20

Pre-gastrointestinal bleeding; rule out ulcers

Post-upper gastrointestinal bleeding; stomach and duodenum appear unremarkable

MEDS:

Demerol 50 mg IV

Versed 3 mg IV

PROCEDURE: Esophagogastroduodenoscopy

The patient was sedated and the scope inserted into the hypopharynx. There was fresh blood oozing from an area in the hiatal hernia pouch just below the gastroesophageal junction. The scope was passed further down to visualize the remainder of the stomach and the duodenum. All areas appeared unremarkable with no other ulcers or lesions identified. The patient tolerated the procedure well. He did have some retching and vomiting after the scope was removed.

CARDIAC CATHERIZATION SUMMARY—PATIENT 13

DATE: 4/19

PROCEDURE:

Left heart catheterization

Left ventricular angiography

Coronary angiography

Stent to mid right coronary artery

After obtaining informed consent the patient was taken to the cardiac catheterization laboratory. He was prepped and draped in the usual fashion and 2% Xylocaine was used to anesthetize the right groin. 6-French sheaths were introduced into the right femoral artery and vein and a 6-French multipurpose catheter was used for left heart catheterization, coronary angiography and left ventricular angiography. I then proceeded to perform a Stent/PTCA to the mid RCA. A HTF wire was used to cross the RCA stenosis and a 4.0-mm J&J Stent was placed in the mid right coronary artery with excellent results. The final angiogram was obtained and the guiding catheterization was removed. The sheaths were securely sutured and the patient tolerated the procedure well without complications.

FINDINGS:

1. Left heart catheterization revealed an elevated resting left ventricular end-diastolic pressure of 18 mm Hg.
2. Left ventricular angiography revealed mild to moderate inferior wall hypokinesis with overall mildly depressed left ventricular systolic function and an estimated global ejection fraction of 45%.
3. Coronary angiography (using single catheter): The left coronary artery arises normally from the left sinus of Valsalva. The left main artery, left anterior descending coronary artery and its branches, and the circumflex artery and its branches have minimal irregularities.

The right coronary artery arises normally from the right sinus of Valsalva. There is a 99% very eccentric stenosis in the large mid right coronary artery and a 70% stenosis of the distal right coronary artery.

IMPRESSION: Arteriosclerotic coronary artery disease was found. There was a successful implantation of 4.0-mm J&J stent in the mid right coronary artery. This site was predilated with a 4.0-mm balloon, then followed by the insertion of a stent.

The mid right coronary artery shows excellent results. Pending the patient's progress we may have to proceed with CABG. The patient will remain on aspirin, Coumadin, and nitrates in the hospital. He will remain on intravenous heparin while his PT levels are adjusted.

LABORATORY REPORTS—PATIENT 13

HEMATOLOGY

DATE: 4/19

Specimen	Results	Normal Values
WBC	9.3	4.3-11.0
RBC	4.4 L	4.5-5.9
HGB	12.7 L	13.5-17.5
HCT	41	41-52
MCV	89	80-100
MCHC	33.9	31-57
PLT	Adequate	150-450

HEMATOLOGY

DATE: 4/20

Specimen	Results	Normal Values
WBC	7.7	4.3-11.0
RBC	4.4 L	4.5-5.9
HGB	12.0 L	13.5-17.5
HCT	41	41-52
MCV	89.6	80-100
MCHC	33.9	31-57
PLT	Adequate	150-450

HEMATOLOGY

DATE: 4/21

Specimen	Results	Normal Values
WBC	8.0	4.3-11.0
RBC	2.88 L	4.5-5.9
HGB	8.6 L	13.5-17.5
HCT	25.8 L	41-52
MCV	89	80-100
MCHC	33.9	31-57
PLT	Adequate	150-450

HEMATOLOGY

DATE: 4/21

Specimen	Results	Normal Values
WBC	8.0	4.3-11.0
RBC	4.5	4.5-5.9
HGB	9.0 L	13.5-17.5
HCT	26.5 L	41-52
MCV	89	80-100
MCHC	33.9	31-57
PLT	Adequate	150-450

HEMATOLOGY

DATE: 4/21

Specimen	Results	Normal Values
WBC	8.0	4.3-11.0
RBC	4.5	4.5-5.9
HGB	9.3 L	13.5-17.5
HCT	27.3 L	41-52
MCV	89	80-100
MCHC	33.9	31-57
PLT	Adequate	150-450

HEMATOLOGY

DATE: 4/22

Specimen	Results	Normal Values
WBC	7.0	4.3-11.0
RBC	2.95 L	4.5-5.9
HGB	9.0 L	13.5-17.5
HCT	26.3 L	41-52
MCV	89	80-100
MCHC	33.9	31-57
PLT	Adequate	150-450

HEMATOLOGY

DATE: 4/23

Specimen	Results	Normal Values
WBC	6.7	4.3-11.0
RBC	2.78 L	4.5-5.9
HGB	8.4 L	13.5-17.5
HCT	24.8 L	41-52
MCV	89.2	80-100
MCHC	34	31-57
PLT	Adequate	150-450

HEMATOLOGY

DATE: 4/24

Specimen	Results	Normal Values
WBC	8.0	4.3-11.0
RBC	4.3 L	4.5-5.9
HGB	9.2 L	13.5-17.5
HCT	27.0 L	41-52
MCV	89	80-100
MCHC	33.9	31-57
PLT	Adequate	150-450

HEMATOLOGY

DATE: 4/25

Specimen	Results	Normal Values
WBC	8.0	4.3-11.0
RBC	4.5	4.5-5.9
HGB	11.1 L	13.5-17.5
HCT	32 L	41-52
MCV	89	80-100
MCHC	33.9	31-57
PLT	Adequate	150-450

LABORATORY REPORTS—PATIENT 13

CHEMISTRY

DATE: 4/19

Specimen	Results	Normal Values
GLUC	97	70–110
BUN	12	8–25
CREAT	1.0	0.5–1.5
NA	134 L	136–146
K	4.0	3.5–5.5
CL	109	95–110
CO_2	33 H	24–32
CA	9.1	8.4–10.5
PHOS	3.0	2.5–4.4
MG	2.0	1.6–3.0
CK	1,702 H	38–120
LD	327 H	106–270
CK MB	93.7 H	0.0–3.0
Relative Index	5.5	
AST	36	0–40
ALT	44	30–65
GCT	70	15–85
LD	110	100–190
ALK PHOS	114	50–136
URIC ACID	6.0	2.2–7.7
CHOL	275 H	0–200
TRIG	140	10–160

CHEMISTRY

DATE: 4/20

Specimen	Results	Normal Values
GLUC	97	70-110
BUN	12	8-25
CREAT	1.0	0.5-1.5
NA	134 L	136-146
K	5.6 H	3.5-5.5
CL	109	95-110
CO_2	33 H	24-32
CA	9.1	8.4-10.5
PHOS	3.0	2.5-4.4
MG	2.0	1.6-3.0
CK	1,277 H	26-221
LD	345 H	106-210
CK MB	68.7 H	0.0-4.4
Relative Index	5.4	
AST	36	0-40
ALT	44	30-65
GCT	70	15-85
LD	110	100-190
ALK PHOS	114	50-136
URIC ACID	6.0	2.2-7.7
CHOL	275 H	0-200
TRIG	140	10-160

CHEMISTRY

DATE: 4/21

Specimen	Results	Normal Values
GLUC	97	70–110
BUN	12	8-25
CREAT	1.0	0.5-1.5
NA	134 L	136-146
K	5.6 H	3.5-5.5
CL	109	95-110
CO_2	33 H	24-32
CA	9.1	8.4-10.5
PHOS	3.0	2.5-4.4
MG	2.0	1.6-3.0
CK	1024 H	26-221
LD	372 H	106-210
CK MB	40.3 H	0.0-4.4
Relative Index	3.9	
AST	36	0-40
ALT	44	30-65
GCT	70	15-85
LD	110	100-190
ALK PHOS	114	50-136
URIC ACID	6.0	2.2-7.7
CHOL	275 H	0-200
TRIG	140	10-160

RADIOLOGY REPORT—PATIENT 13

DATE: 4/19

CHEST, SUPINE: There is no gross evidence of acute inflammatory disease or congestive heart failure.

IMPRESSION: No acute disease.

RADIOLOGY REPORT—PATIENT 13

DATE: 4/21

DIAGNOSIS: The patient appears to have undergone sternotomy. The heart appears normal. The endotracheal tube is in place as is the Swan-Ganz catheter.

IMPRESSION: Stable postoperative chest

EKG REPORT—PATIENT 13

DATE: 4/19

IMPRESSION: Elevated ST changes. Cannot eliminate the possibility of ischemia. Complete heart block is also noted.

EKG REPORT—PATIENT 13

DATE: 4/20

IMPRESSION: Acute inferior myocardial infarction. Complete heart block has resolved.

Enter nine diagnosis codes and eleven procedure codes.

PDX

DX2

DX3

DX4

DX5

DX6

DX7

DX8

DX9

PP1

PR2

PR3

PR4

PR5

PR6

PR7

PR8

PR9

PR10

PR11

CCS
Practice Exam 2

A blank answer sheet for these multiple choice questions can be found on page 169.

Domain 1: Health Information Documentation

1. A 23-year-old female is admitted for vaginal bleeding following a miscarriage two weeks prior to this admission. She is afebrile at this time and is treated with an aspiration dilation and curettage. Products of conception are found. Which of the following should be the principal diagnosis?
   a. 634.11, Spontaneous abortion complicated by delayed or excessive hemorrhage, incomplete
   b. 639.1, Complication following abortion and ectopic and molar pregnancies, delayed or excessive hemorrhage
   c. 785.50, Shock, unspecified
   d. 998.0, Postoperative shock

2. A psychiatrist documents that a patient has wide mood swings from excessive happiness to loss of energy and crying. What condition is suspected?
   a. Bipolar disorder
   b. Major depression
   c. Anxiety
   d. Psychosis

3. A patient with a cephalic presentation anticipating a vaginal delivery failed to progress. After measurement of the fetal head and a trial of oxytocin, the patient underwent a cesarean section. What condition should the coder suspect and query the physician about?
   a. Twin pregnancy
   b. Early delivery
   c. Eclampsia
   d. Cephalopelvic disproportion

4. A 45-year-old woman underwent a carotid bypass and experienced a significant drop in blood pressure during the surgery about which documentation suggested the patient may have had a myocardial infarction. In accordance with coding guidelines, what should the coding professional do?
   a. Code complication of surgery NOS.
   b. Query the physician to determine if the patient had hypertension.
   c. Query the physician to determine if there was a complication of surgery.
   d. Code preoperative shock.

5. If a patient's discharge summary does not contain a given condition that is documented by the anesthesiologist in a preoperative evaluation and that would impact MS-DRG assignment, the coder should:
   a. Code only from the discharge diagnoses.
   b. Code the diagnosis reflected on the anesthesia preoperative evaluation.
   c. Code the most severe symptom.
   d. Query the attending physician regarding the clinical significance of that diagnosis

6. A patient has documentation of esophageal varices. What condition may be related that may affect coding?
   a. Arthritis
   b. Liver disease
   c. Chronic obstructive pulmonary disease
   d. Erythema

7. A patient admitted with acute abdominal pain, is found to have appendicitis, and has an appendectomy. The patient has a length of stay of 2 days. What type of patient encounter is this?
   a. Inpatient
   b. Outpatient
   c. Long-term care
   d. Rehabilitation

8. A patient is treated in the emergency department for a swollen knee for which an aspiration of the joint was performed. The patient was then discharged home. It is important to make sure that which of the following are documented and captured for billing purposes?
   a. X-rays and other types of radiology examinations
   b. Procedures performed including the aspiration of the joint
   c. Examination and management in the emergency department
   d. All services provided including diagnostic and treatment procedures, as well as physician services

9. A patient has documentation on the discharge summary of urosepsis. The coding staff queries the attending physician about the condition and is provided further information that the patient has septicemia. This is in alignment with the laboratory tests and medication given but the diagnosis of septicemia was not documented by the physician. How should the physician be requested to document the septicemia?

   a. A brand new history and physical should be dictated to replace the one in the record.

   b. An addendum to the chart should be written.

   c. The new information should be squeezed in between lines within the progress notes of the last day.

   d. The query sheet will be sufficient to document this information.

Domain 2: Diagnosis Coding

10. An inpatient is discharged with a diagnosis of "abdominal pain, rule out irritable bowel syndrome vs. pancreatitis." The coder would code which condition as the principal diagnosis?

    a. Abdominal pain

    b. Abdominal pain and irritable bowel syndrome

    c. Irritable bowel syndrome

    d. Observation for suspected gastrointestinal condition

11. A 55-year-old male was transferred to a nursing home for continuing care due to being placed on mechanical ventilation following complications of cardiac bypass surgery. He was readmitted three weeks later due to ventilator associated pneumonia (VAP) due to pseudomonas aeruginosa. How should this be coded?

    a. 999.9, 486, 041.7

    b. 483.8

    c. 997.31, 041.7

    d. 482.1, 997.31

12. A patient takes Coumadin as prescribed, and it is correctly administered. However, the patient develops hematuria due to the Coumadin. The correct coding assignment for this case would be:

    a. Poisoning due to Coumadin

    b. Unspecified adverse reaction to Coumadin

    c. Hematuria, poisoning due to Coumadin

    d. Hematuria, adverse reaction to Coumadin

13. A patient is admitted with lethargy, congestive heart failure, and pleural effusion. The patient underwent treatment with diuretics for the CHF, which has cleared. The pleural effusion required a thoracentesis to determine the cause. At the time of discharge, the effusion was decreased but not resolved. The correct coding assignment for this case would be:

    a. Congestive heart failure
    b. Pleural effusion
    c. Both congestive heart failure and pleural effusion
    d. Lethargy, congestive heart failure, and pleural effusion

14. A patient with human immunodeficiency virus (HIV) with methicillin susceptible pneumonia due to staphylococcus aureus was discharged from the acute-care setting. How should this be coded?

042	Human immunodeficiency virus (HIV) disease
482.40	Pneumonia due to staphylococcus, unspecified
482.41	Methicillin susceptible pneumonia due to staphylococcus aureus
482.42	Methicillin resistant pneumonia due to staphylococcus aureus
484.8	Pneumonia in other infectious diseases classified elsewhere

    a. 042, 484.8
    b. 042, 482.40
    c. 042, 482.41
    d. 042, 482.42

15. A patient has a diabetic ulcer of the right heel. How should this patient's record be coded?

250.00	Diabetes mellitus without mention of complication, type II or unspecified type, not stated as uncontrolled
250.01	Diabetes mellitus without mention of complication, type I [juvenile type], not stated as uncontrolled
250.02	Diabetes mellitus without mention of complication, type II or unspecified type, uncontrolled
250.03	Diabetes mellitus without mention of complication, type I [juvenile type], uncontrolled
250.60	Diabetes with neurological manifestations, type II or unspecified type, not stated as uncontrolled
250.61	Diabetes with neurological manifestations, type I [juvenile type], not stated as uncontrolled
250.62	Diabetes with neurological manifestations, type II or unspecified type, uncontrolled
250.63	Diabetes with neurological manifestations, type I [juvenile type], uncontrolled
250.70	Diabetes with peripheral circulatory disorders, type II or unspecified type, not stated as uncontrolled
250.71	Diabetes with peripheral circulatory disorders, type I [juvenile type], not stated as uncontrolled
250.72	Diabetes with peripheral circulatory disorders, type II or unspecified type, uncontrolled
250.73	Diabetes with peripheral circulatory disorders, type I [juvenile type], uncontrolled
250.80	Diabetes with other specified manifestations, type II or unspecified type, not stated as uncontrolled
250.81	Diabetes with other specified manifestations, type I [juvenile type], not stated as uncontrolled
250.82	Diabetes with other specified manifestations, type II or unspecified type, uncontrolled
250.83	Diabetes with other specified manifestations, type I [juvenile type], uncontrolled
707.14	Ulcer of lower limbs, except pressure ulcer, ulcer of heel and midfoot

a. 250.00, 707.14

b. 250.60, 707.14

c. 250.70, 707.14

d. 250.80, 707.14

16. Assign code(s) for the following diagnosis: Congestive heart failure due to hypertension.

401.9	Essential hypertension, unspecified
402.90	Hypertensive heart disease, unspecified, without heart failure
402.91	Hypertensive heart disease, unspecified, with heart failure
428.0	Congestive heart failure, unspecified
428.1	Left heart failure
428.20	Systolic heart failure, unspecified
428.21	Systolic heart failure, acute
428.22	Systolic heart failure, chronic
428.23	Systolic heart failure, acute on chronic

a. 401.9, 428.0

b. 402.91

c. 428.23, 401.9

d. 402.91, 428.0

17. A patient has squamous cell carcinoma of the knee. What code should be assigned for this diagnosis?

171.3	Malignant neoplasm of connective and other soft tissue, lower limb, including hip
172.7	Malignant melanoma of skin of lower limb, including hip
173.7	Malignant neoplasm of skin, skin of lower limb, including hip
195.5	Malignant neoplasm of other and ill-defined sites, lower limb

a. 171.3

b. 172.7

c. 173.7

d. 195.5

18. A patient is seen for evaluation of a right orbital roof fracture. How should this be coded?

801.00	Fracture of base of skull, closed without mention of intracranial injury, unspecified state of consciousness
802.6	Fracture of face bones, orbital floor (blow-out), closed
802.8	Fracture of face bones, other facial bones, closed
803.0	Other and unqualified skull fractures, closed without mention of intracranial injury

a. 801.00

b. 802.6

c. 802.8

d. 803.0

19. A patient was seen for first- and second-degree burns of the upper thigh. How should this be coded?

945.09	Burn of lower limb(s), unspecified degree, lower limb (leg), unspecified site
945.06	Burn of lower limb(s), unspecified degree, thigh [any part]
945.16	Burn of lower limb(s), erythema [first degree], thigh [any part]
945.26	Burn of lower limb(s), blisters, epidermal loss [second degree], thigh [any part]

a. 945.09

b. 945.06

c. 945.16, 945.26

d. 945.26

20. Suicide attempt with overdose of Percocet. How should this be coded?

305.50	Abuse of opioid, unspecified
965.09	Poisoning by opiates and related narcotics, other
E935.2	Adverse effect in therapeutic use of other opiates and related narcotics
E950.0	Suicide and self-inflicted poisoning by analgesics, antipyretics, and antirheumatics
E980.0	Poisoning by solid or liquid substances, undetermined whether accidentally or purposefully inflicted, analgesics, antipyretics, and antirheumatics

a. 305.50, E950.0

b. 965.09, E950.0

c. 305.50, E935.2

d. 965.09, E980.0

21. Drug reaction to an antihistamine taken at home and prescribed correctly by the physician in his office. What codes should be assigned?

796.0	Nonspecific abnormal toxicological findings
995.20	Unspecified adverse effect of unspecified drug, medicinal and biological substance
963.0	Poisoning by antiallergic and antiemetic drugs
E933.0	Adverse effect of antiallergic and antiemetic drugs
E980.4	Poisoning by solid or liquid substances, undetermined whether accidentally or purposefully inflicted, analgesics, other specified drugs and medicinal substances

a. 796.0, 963.0

b. 796.0, E933.0

c. 995.20, 963.0

d. 995.20, E933.0

Domain 3: Procedure Coding

22. Assign the best answer to complete the following sentence. The CPT codes for treatment of fractures:

a. Use the terminology "manipulation" rather than "reduction" of fracture.

b. Include internal fixation in all codes.

c. Do not include application of cast.

d. Do not differentiate between open and closed treatment; CPT only specifies the site of the fracture.

23. In CPT, if a patient has two lacerations of the arm that are repaired with simple closures, the coder would assign:

a. Two CPT codes expressing each laceration repair

b. One CPT code for the largest laceration

c. One CPT code, adding the lengths of the lacerations together

d. One CPT code for the most complex closure

24. According to CPT, a repair of a laceration that includes retention sutures would be considered what type of closure?

a. Simple

b. Intermediate

c. Not specified

d. Complex

25. The patient was monitored under general anesthesia for keratoplasty including excision of diseased cornea. A controlled depth-setting blade was used to cut partially into the recipient's cornea in a manner to allow the lamellar graft to fit. Which CPT code should be assigned?

65710	Keratoplasty (corneal transplant); anterior lamellar
65730	Keratoplasty (corneal transplant); penetrating (except in aphakia or pseudophakia)
65750	Keratoplasty (corneal transplant); penetrating (in aphakia)
65755	Keratoplasty (corneal transplant); penetrating (in pseudophakia)

a. 65710

b. 65730

c. 65750

d. 65755

26. Assign the correct CPT code for a 50-year-old female patient admitted to outpatient surgery department for laparoscopic surgical repair of a recurrent, incarcerated incisional hernia with mesh insertion.

49561	Repair initial incisional or ventral hernia; incarcerated or strangulated
49566	Repair recurrent incisional or ventral hernia; incarcerated or strangulated
49657	Laparoscopy, surgical, repair, recurrent incisional hernia (includes mesh insertion, when performed); incarcerated or strangulated
49565	Repair recurrent incisional or ventral hernia, reducible

a. 49561

b. 49566

c. 49657

d. 49565

27. Patient with renal tumors received percutaneous cryotherapy ablation of three tumors on the right kidney in the same operative episode at Memorial Hospital. Assign a CPT code for this procedure.

50592	Ablation, 1 or more renal tumor(s), percutaneous, unilateral, radiofrequency
50593	Ablation, renal tumor(s), unilateral, percutaneous, cryotherapy
50590	Lithotripsy, extracorporeal shock wave
50250	Ablation, open, 1 or more renal mass lesion(s), cryosurgical, including intraoperative ultrasound guidance and monitoring, if performed

a. 50592

b. 50593

c. 50590

d. 50250

28. In outpatient surgery, a PTCA is completed with insertion of a drug-eluting stent in the left circumflex artery and a non-drug-eluting stent inserted into the left anterior descending artery of this 56-year-old female. Assign the correct CPT code(s) for this procedure.

92980	Transcatheter placement of an intracoronary stent(s), percutaneous, with or without other therapeutic intervention, any method; single vessel
92981	Transcatheter placement of an intracoronary stent(s), percutaneous, with or without other therapeutic intervention, any method; each additional vessel (List separately in addition to code for primary procedure.)
G0290	Transcatheter placement of a drug eluting intracoronary stent(s), percutaneous, with or without other therapeutic intervention, any method; single vessel
G0291	Transcatheter placement of a drug eluting intracoronary stent(s), percutaneous, with or without other therapeutic intervention, any method; each additional vessel
-LC	Left circumflex coronary artery
-LD	Left anterior descending coronary artery

a. 92981–LC, 92980–LD

b. 92980–LC, 92981–LD

c. G0291–LC, 92980–LD

d. G0290–LC, 92981–LD

29. Patient admitted for laparoscopic repair of diaphragmatic hernia via abdominal approach. Assign the ICD-9-CM procedure code for this surgery.

53.71	Laparoscopic repair of diaphragmatic hernia, abdominal approach
53.72	Other and open repair of diaphragmatic hernia, abdominal approach
53.83	Laparoscopic repair of diaphragmatic hernia, with thoracic approach
53.84	Other and open repair of diaphragmatic hernia, with thoracic approach

a. 53.71

b. 53.72

c. 53.83

d. 53.84

30. Patient presents in the ER with thrombosis of a loop PTFE hemodialysis fistula without mechanical complications. The physician performed a thrombectomy of the left forearm graft. Assign a facility code for this outpatient procedure.

39.49	Other revision of vascular procedure
36831	Thrombectomy, open, arteriovenous fistula without revision, autogenous or nonautogenous dialysis graft (separate procedure)
36832	Revision, open, arteriovenous fistula; without thrombectomy, autogenous or nonautogenous dialysis graft (separate procedure)
37184	Primary percutaneous transluminal mechanical thrombectomy, noncoronary, arterial or arterial bypass graft, including fluoroscopic guidance and intraprocedural pharmacological thrombolytic injection(s); initial vessel

a. 39.49

b. 36831

c. 37184

d. 36832

31. Physician performed a myringotomy under general anesthesia for insertion of ventilating tubes bilaterally on a 4-year-old male due to chronic otitis media as an outpatient procedure. What is the CPT code assignment and what modifier should be appended (if applicable) to this procedure code?

69421	Myringotomy including aspiration and/or eustachian tube inflation requiring general anesthesia
69436	Tympanostomy (requiring insertion of ventilating tube), general anesthesia
-50	Bilateral procedure
-51	Multiple procedures
-RT	Right side
-LT	Left side

a. 69421–RT

b. 69421–LT

c. 69436–51

d. 69436–50

32. Removal of two (2) skin tags on chest (0.3 cm and 0.5 cm). What is the correct CPT code(s) assignment?

11200	Removal of skin tags, multiple fibrocutaneous tags, any area; up to and including 15 lesions
11201	Removal of skin tags, multiple fibrocutaneous tags, any area;each additional 10 lesions, or part thereof (List separately in additional to code for primary procedure.)
11305	Shaving of epidermal or dermal lesion, single lesion, scalp neck, hands, feet, genitalia; lesion diameter 0.5 cm or less

a. 11200, 11201

b. 11305, 11305

c. 11305

d. 11200

Domain 4: Regulatory Guidelines and Reporting Requirements for Acute-Care (Inpatient) Service

33. According to the UHDDS, the definition of a *secondary diagnosis* is a condition that:
    a. Is recorded in the patient record
    b. Receives evaluation and is documented by the physician
    c. Receives clinical evaluation, therapeutic treatment, further evaluation, extends the length of stay, increases nursing monitoring/care
    d. Is considered to be essential by the physicians involved and is reflected in the record

34. A female patient is diagnosed with congestive heart failure and also has a stage IV pressure ulcer. Which of the following indicators must be present so that the ulcer will be classified as a MCC for this admission?
    a. N
    b. Y
    c. W
    d. U

35. A patient is admitted to a healthcare facility with ataxia and syncope. The patient has a history of lung cancer. The patient also has a fractured arm as a result of falling. The patient undergoes a closed reduction of the fracture in the emergency department and a complete workup for metastatic carcinoma of the brain. The patient is found to have metastatic carcinoma of the lung to the brain and undergoes radiation therapy to the brain. The principal diagnosis should be:
    a. Fractured arm
    b. Syncope
    c. Metastatic carcinoma of the brain
    d. Carcinoma of the lung

36. A 78-year-old patient is admitted with shortness of breath and a chest x-ray reveals infiltrates in the lung with pleural effusion. The patient also has a history of hypertension with left ventricular hypertrophy. The patient is given Lasix and the shortness of breath is relieved. From the information given, what is the probable principal diagnosis?
    a. Pneumonia
    b. Congestive heart failure
    c. Pleural effusion
    d. Chronic obstructive pulmonary disease

37. A patient is admitted with abdominal pain. The discharge documentation specifies "pancreatitis vs. noncalculus cholecystitis" as the final diagnoses. Both diagnoses are equally treated. Based on coding guidelines, the correct conditions that could be assigned codes and the sequencing for them in this case would be:
    a. Sequence either the pancreatitis or noncalculus cholecystitis first
    b. Pancreatitis; noncalculus cholecystitis; abdominal pain
    c. Noncalculus cholecystitis; pancreatitis
    d. Sequence the abdominal pain first, followed by pancreatitis and noncalculus cholecystitis as secondary diagnoses

38. A patient undergoes a procedure and has a postoperative complication. The insurance company will not pay for the entire amount requested. Which POA indicator is likely part of the cause?
    a. N
    b. Y
    c. W
    d. U

Domain 5: Regulatory Guidelines and Reporting Requirements for Outpatient Services

39. Which of the following is *not* a function of the outpatient code editor (OCE)?
    a. Editing the data on the claim for accuracy
    b. Specifying the action the FI should take when specific edits occur
    c. Assigning APCs to the claim (for hospital outpatient services)
    d. Determining payment-related conditions that require direct reference to ICD-9-CM codes

40. According to CPT guidelines, a colonoscopy includes:
    a. Examination of the rectum and sigmoid colon
    b. Examination of the entire rectum, sigmoid colon, and may include examination of a portion of the descending colon
    c. Examination of the entire colon from the rectum to the cecum
    d. Examination of the entire colon, from the rectum to the cecum, and may include the examination of the terminal ileum

41. A female patient with hematochezia presents to the hospital outpatient surgery department for a colonoscopy but the procedure was not performed due to elevated blood pressure. What is the first-listed diagnosis for this encounter?

    a. Elevated blood pressure

    b. Hematochezia

    c. Procedure not performed due to contraindication

    d. Procedure not performed for other reason

Use the information in this table to answer questions 42 through 44.

Billing Number	Status Indicator	CPT/HCPCS	APC	Reimbursement*
989323	T	10060	0006	$500
989323	T	64605	0220	$1,000
989323	X	71010	0260	$50.00
989323	S	38230	0112	$2,000

**This is not the actual reimbursement for the designated APC.*

42. From the information provided, what would be the total reimbursement for this patient?

    a. $3,550

    b. $3,000

    c. $3,050

    d. $3,300

43. What percentage will the facility be paid for procedure code 10060?

    a. 50%

    b. 75%

    c. 0%

    d. 100%

44. If another status S procedure were performed, how much would the facility receive for the second status S procedure?

    a. 50%

    b. 75%

    c. 0%

    d. 100%

Domain 6: Data Quality and Management

45. Which of the following services are paid under the outpatient prospective payment system (OPPS)?

    a. Ambulance services

    b. Outpatient hernia repair

    c. Clinical diagnostic laboratory test performed on the same day as a surgical procedure

    d. Inpatient procedures

46. What is assigned to CPT codes to indicate whether a service or procedure will be reimbursed under the OPPS?

    a. Ambulatory payment classifications

    b. Payment status indicators

    c. Payment modifiers

    d. Diagnosis-related groups

47. Diagnostic-related groups (DRGs) and ambulatory patient classifications (APCs) are dissimilar in that:

    a. There is only one MS-DRG per inpatient visit with one or more APCs per outpatient visit

    b. There are many MS-DRGs per inpatient visit with only one APC per outpatient visit

    c. There are more possible MS-DRGs for inpatients that there are APCs for outpatients

    d. There are up to three MS-DRGs per each inpatient visit while there are only up to seven APCs per outpatient visit

Refer to the following data when answering questions 48 and 49. (*Note:* The DRG numbers and weights are not actual numbers and weights for fiscal year 2011.)

MS-DRG	MS-DRG Wt.	Number of Patients
191	2.0	10
192	1.5	10
193	1.0	10

48. The case mix for the information provided above is:

    a. 30

    b. 20

    c. 45

    d. 15

49. The information provided shows that:

    a. The payment is lowest for patients with DRG 193.

    b. There are more patients with DRG 191.

    c. The case-mix index could decrease if more patients in DRG 191 were admitted.

    d. The case-mix index would increase if more patients in DRG 193 were admitted.

Domain 7: Information and Communication Technologies

50. The quality management director is working on physician reappointment reports and needs to focus on all physicians who attended patients with pneumonia during the last quarter. She asks the coder to get a list of all pneumonia patients who did not have an x-ray done during their stay. To perform this task efficiently, the coder should do the following: (Note: The same time frame applies to all reports.)

    a. Obtain a list of all patients whose principal diagnosis was pneumonia, retrieve those patient records, and look for documentation of the x-ray. Upon finding, record the patient information and attending physician.

    b. Obtain a list of all patients whose DRG was simple pneumonia and pleurisy, retrieve those patient records, and identify documentation of x-ray and physician responsible.

    c. Obtain a list of all patients who were diagnosed with pneumonia, retrieve those patient records, identify patients who did not have an x-ray done along with the physician responsible, and record this information in a spreadsheet.

    d. Obtain a list of all patients who were diagnosed with pneumonia, retrieve a list of all patients who had an x-ray from the charge master, compare both lists, and identify patients who did not have an x-ray along with the physician responsible.

51. The blood usage review committee is trying to identify physicians who have ordered blood transfusion without following the predetermined criteria during the last quarter. How can this be done most efficiently?

    a. Obtain a list of all blood transfusions given in the facility during the quarter along with the ordering physician, manually identify cases with the highest amount of packed cells received, retrieve those patient records, and determine whether the criteria was followed.

    b. Obtain a list of all blood transfusions given in the facility during the designated quarter along with the ordering physicians and lab values for RBC. Import the list into a spreadsheet and sort the data by the highest blood transfusion amount.

    c. Obtain a list of all blood transfusions given in the facility during the designated quarter along with the ordering physicians and lab values for RBC. Import the list in a spreadsheet and sort the data by the highest RBC value.

    d. Obtain a list of all blood transfusions given in the facility during the designated quarter along with the ordering physicians and lab values for RBC. Import the list into a spreadsheet and filter the data by using the RBC predetermined values or lower in the facility criteria for blood transfusion.

52. A quality improvement study showed that maternity cases are not being coded with the correct procedure code for manually assisted vaginal delivery codes associated. What HIM software could be used to evaluate this?

    a. Birth certificate registry or master patient index

    b. Transcription registry or correspondence registry

    c. Quality improvement or operative registry

    d. Billing and reimbursement abstracting system

Domain 8: Privacy, Confidentiality, Legal, and Ethical Issues

53. According to the AHIMA Standards of Ethical Coding, "A coder should protect the confidentiality of the health record at all times and refuse to access protected health information not required for coding-related activities." Which of the following is *not* considered a coding-related activity?

    a. Coding quality evaluation

    b. Review of records assigned each day

    c. Risk analysis of medical record documentation

    d. Completion of abstracting

54. A routine computer back-up procedure is an example of a control that ensures data loss does not occur. This type of control is:

    a. Computer
    b. Validity
    c. Responsive
    d. Preventive

55. The patient was admitted for prostate carcinoma. This was treated with radiation. A member of the medical staff who was not associated with the patient's care requests to see the patient's record. What should the coder do?

    a. Provide the record to the physician.
    b. Report the incident to hospital security.
    c. Ask the physician to come back when the supervisor gets back.
    d. Explain that providing the record would violate the privacy policy.

56. The billing department has requested that a copy of the operative report be provided when unlisted CPT codes are used. The coding staff should:

    a. Provide the report because insurers will not provide reimbursement without this documentation.
    b. Not provide the report.
    c. Require patient consent for this specific type of release.
    d. Ignore the request.

Domain 9: Compliance

57. According to Medicare requirements, a history and physical must:

    a. Be coded based on the uniform hospital discharge proposal
    b. Include the patient's weight, height, body mass index, and year of birth
    c. Be completed for each patient no more than 30 days before or 24 hours after admission or registration, but prior to surgery
    d. Discuss the educational plans for the patient including diet, exercise, and plans for smoking cessation

58. Which of the following is an important part of a coding compliance plan for facility-based evaluation and management code assignment?

    a. Regular internal audits comparing the code assignment to the facility guidelines
    b. Audits performed by objective external reviewers
    c. Coding audits performed by physician payers
    d. Sharing and discussing results with admission staff

59. Proper discharge planning for inpatients being transferred to another healthcare delivery system must include a complete summary of the patient's history, current status, and future needs to ensure appropriate:

    a. Coding
    b. Billing
    c. Continuity of care
    d. Quality of care

60. Which of the following is *not* part of a coding compliance plan?

    a. Regular internal audits
    b. Audits performed by objective external reviewers
    c. Coding audits performed by payers
    d. Sharing and discussing results with coding staff

Multiple Choice Practice Exam 2 Answers

1. __________
2. __________
3. __________
4. __________
5. __________
6. __________
7. __________
8. __________
9. __________
10. __________
11. __________
12. __________
13. __________
14. __________
15. __________
16. __________
17. __________
18. __________
19. __________
20. __________
21. __________
22. __________
23. __________
24. __________
25. __________
26. __________
27. __________
28. __________
29. __________
30. __________
31. __________
32. __________
33. __________
34. __________
35. __________
36. __________
37. __________
38. __________
39. __________
40. __________
41. __________
42. __________
43. __________
44. __________
45. __________
46. __________
47. __________
48. __________
49. __________
50. __________
51. __________
52. __________
53. __________
54. __________
55. __________
56. __________
57. __________
58. __________
59. __________
60. __________

CCS
Practice Exam 2
Case Studies

Note: Review the Coding Instructions (for the Exam) in the Introduction of this book.

SAME DAY SURGERY RECORD—PATIENT 1

DATE OF ADMISSION: 1/29 **DATE OF DISCHARGE:** 1/29

DISCHARGE DIAGNOSIS: Torn lateral meniscus of the right knee; torn anterior cruciate ligament of the right knee

ADMISSION HISTORY: The patient is a 17-year-old male who approximately 1 year ago underwent a cruciate ligament reconstruction. He has had several reinjuries and for this reason was taken for arthroscopic evaluation and treatment.

COURSE IN HOSPITAL: The patient was taken to the OR where a resection of tear of the lateral meniscus posterior horn and reconstruction of the anterior cruciate ligament using patellar tendon graft was performed. The patient was then discharged and asked to return in 1 week.

INSTRUCTIONS ON DISCHARGE:
Levaquin 500 mg by mouth, 1 per day
Tylox 1–2 capsules as needed for pain
Follow-up appointment in 1 week

HISTORY AND PHYSICAL EXAMINATION—PATIENT 1

DATE: 1/29

HISTORY OF PRESENT ILLNESS: This is a 17-year-old male active in several sports. He then reinjured the knee several times this year while playing soccer.

PAST MEDICAL HISTORY: The patient has no other health problems.

ALLERGIES: None known

CHRONIC MEDICATIONS: None

FAMILY HISTORY: Noncontributory

PHYSICAL EXAMINATION: Reveals a well-developed, well-nourished white male in no apparent distress. HEENT reveals nothing abnormal. Chest was clear to auscultation and percussion. Heart sounds were normal with no murmurs. Examination of the abdomen reveals no masses or tenderness. Examination of the genitals was not done. Examination of the extremities reveals a scar on the left knee with swelling of the joint. Distal sensation and circulation were normal.

IMPRESSION: Torn lateral meniscus of the right knee; torn anterior cruciate ligament of the right knee.

PLAN:
1. Resection of tear of the lateral meniscus posterior horn.
2. Reconstruction of the anterior cruciate ligament using patellar tendon graft

PROGRESS NOTES—PATIENT 1

DATE	NOTE
1/29	Admit to Same Day Surgery unit
	Prep for surgery
	Betadine scrub right leg
	Demerol 100 mg IM 1 hr preop
	Versed 5 mg IM 1 hr preop
	Postop Orders:
	Demerol 75 mg. PRN pain 1 dose
	Tylox 1 to 2 PO q. 4 hr
	Levaquin 500 mg PO postop
	D/C when stable as per discharge criteria

PHYSICIAN'S ORDERS—PATIENT 1

DATE	ORDER
1/29	Patient admitted for surgical and diagnostic arthroscopy.

Brief OP Note

PREOP DX: Torn lateral meniscus of the right knee; torn anterior cruciate ligament of the right knee.

POSTOP DX: Torn lateral meniscus of the right knee; torn anterior cruciate ligament of the right knee.

OPERATION:

1. Resection of tear of the lateral meniscus posterior horn
2. Reconstruction of the anterior cruciate ligament using patellar tendon graft

ANES: General

Good circulation and sensation. Will encourage patient to ambulate with splint and crutches. Discharge when stable. Follow-up in one week with my office.

DISCHARGE MEDICATIONS:

1. Levaquin 500 mg by mouth, one per day
2. Tylox 1–2 capsules as needed for pain

OPERATIVE REPORT—PATIENT 1

PREOPERATIVE DIAGNOSIS: Torn lateral meniscus of the right knee; torn anterior cruciate ligament of the right knee

POSTOPERATIVE DIAGNOSIS: Torn lateral meniscus of the right knee; torn anterior cruciate ligament of the right knee

OPERATION:
1. Resection of tear of the lateral meniscus posterior horn
2. Reconstruction of the anterior cruciate ligament using patellar tendon graft

ANESTHESIA: General

CLINICAL HISTORY: This is a 17-year-old male who sustained an injury to his right knee in May during a surfing accident. He was treated conservatively before this. But because of instability and pain, he wished to have the following procedure done.
Tourniquet was used for one hour, 50 minutes

PROCEDURE DESCRIPTION: The patient was placed under general anesthesia. Airway was maintained by Dr. Spears, as the right lower limb was manipulated and found to have a positive Lachman, a positive drawer test, and a trace pivot shift. The left knee was also examined and found to have the same findings.

The knee was prepped with a gel prep, draped with the limb free. Tourniquet was applied to the thigh but not elevated to begin with. The procedure done first was a diagnostic arthroscopy and during this, we found that the anterior cruciate ligament was torn away from the wall lateral femoral condyle. It was quite lax as well. Attention was turned to the lateral compartment where the initial look at the lateral cartilage showed that it was fine. But on probing underneath the surface of the posterior horn, there was a partial tear but without any instability. The tear extended through the cartilage 50% to 75%. Because of this, this portion was resected back to normal cartilage, removing the torn segment. This was in an area that was not vascular.

Attention was then turned to the anterior cruciate ligament which was resected. Using a shaver, all the soft tissue was removed from around and up into the notch. A bur was used to enlarge the notch superiorly, into the lateral side and into the depth of the notch to the over-the-top position which was clearly delineated.

OPERATIVE REPORT—PATIENT 1 (continued)

The first part of the arthroscopy was terminated. The tourniquet was elevated. Then an incision was made from the mid patella to the tibial tubercle, with dissection carried down to the patellar tendon. The middle third of the patellar tendon was harvested with bone graft from tibia and fibula which was sized to a 10-rom tunnel size. Two threads were placed in the femoral portion and one in the tibial portion, and the femoral portion marked at the interface between the bone and the tendon. The small saw was used to cut the bone graft from both the tibia and the patella. The patellar defect was filled with bone graft and closed. The guide for the tibial tunnel was then put in place, measuring about 55 degrees. This was placed just in front of the posterior tibial tendon and in the mid portion of the slope of the tibial spine. The guide wire was put in place, found to be satisfactory, and a 10-rom channel was reamed. The over-the-top positioning was put into placed with a guidewire. This was in the eleven o'clock for the right knee. The bulldog cannulated reamer was used, and a footprint was established. Probing revealed there to be a millimeter of bone posterior to this. This was reamed up to 30 mm in size for the graft plus 5 rom. The guidewire was removed. The eccentric guide was put into place, and a notch made. Then the two-pin passer was passed through the eccentric guide, and then the guide was removed. The exit of the two-pin passer was in a proper place on the anterolateral thigh. A guidewire was used to put in place in the two-pin passer, and the graft was passed up into the channel and seemed to fit well. A biodegradable screw was used, but the first one did not cut properly and had to be replaced after tapping the spot for the screw. A second biodegradable screw was put up in place. This was approximately 25 mm × 9 mm. The position and tightness were excellent, and drawer test at this point was trace, as was the Lachman. There was no impingement of the graft with extension, and no change in the length. The screw for the tibia was put into place over a guidewire, and this was an 8 × 25 tibial screw. This again was quite tight, and the Lachman test was just a trace positive.

The joint and the wound were irrigated with arthroscopic fluid, and subcutaneous tissues were closed with 2-0 Vicryl. The skin was closed with 4-0 nylon, as was each of the ports. The incision plus the ports were all injected with 0.25% Marcaine with epinephrine. The patient was given 30 mg of Toradol. Dressing was applied of Xeroform gauze, 4 × 4s, Kerlix, Ace wrap, and then the patient's brace which was a Bledsoe brace.

He tolerated the procedure well with a tourniquet time of 1 hour 50 minutes. Blood loss was nil. He will be sent home on Lortab. He will return to the office on Friday for a dressing change. He will be contacted tomorrow.

PHYSICIAN'S ORDERS—PATIENT 1

DATE	ORDER
4/1/20XX	Attending MD: Admit to same-day surgery Betadine scrub ×3 Preop May take own meds Lasix 20 mg now
4/1/20XX	Anesthesia Note: Continue NPO Demerol 50 mg IM 1½ hr Preop Vistaril 50 mg IM 1½ hr Preop Atropine 0.4 mg IM 1½ hr Preop
4/1/20XX	Attending MD: Vital signs q. 15 min until stable Regular diet Percocet 2.5 mg. q. 4 hrs p.r.n. for pain Iron supplement q.d. for anemia Discharge to home when stable

LABORATORY REPORTS—PATIENT 1

HEMATOLOGY

DATE: 3/31

Specimen	Results	Normal Values
WBC	7.2	4.3-11.0
RBC	4.0 L	4.5-5.9
HGB	11.0 L	13.5-17.5
HCT	38.0 L	41-52
MCV	94	80-100
MCHC	40	31-57
PLT	300	150-400

Enter two diagnosis codes and two procedure codes.

PDX

DX2

PP1

PR2

SAME DAY SURGERY SUMMARY—PATIENT 2

DATE OF ADMISSION: 12/30 **DATE OF DISCHARGE:** 12/30

DISCHARGE DIAGNOSIS: Bunion of 1st metatarsal

ADMISSION HISTORY: This is a 45-year-old white female in good health. Her family physician has performed a history and physical that demonstrated her health is within normal limits. The patient has no known allergies, good pedal pulses. The patient has a bunion of the left 1st metatarsal.

COURSE IN HOSPITAL: The patient was admitted to same-day surgery for osteotomy of the 1st metatarsal. The patient was taken to the OR where this was accomplished. The patient tolerated the procedure well and is discharged to home in stable condition.

INSTRUCTIONS ON DISCHARGE:

Keep foot elevated.

Keep dressing dry; do not change until seen by your physician.

Use surgical shoe.

Take Percocet 2.5 mg every 4 hours as needed for pain.

HISTORY AND PHYSICAL EXAMINATION—PATIENT 2

DATE: 12/30

HISTORY OF PRESENT ILLNESS: The patient has had increased long-term pain with difficulty ambulating.

PAST MEDICAL HISTORY: The patient has no major health problems and has not undergone major surgery.

ALLERGIES: None known

CHRONIC MEDICATIONS: None

FAMILY HISTORY: Noncontributory

PHYSICAL EXAMINATION:

IMPRESSION: B.P. 130/88, pulse is 68, respirations 20, temp 97.3. HEENT, within normal limits. Heart, normal. Lungs, clear. Abdomen, soft with bowel sounds. Pelvic and rectal deferred. Extremities, normal except bunion on 1st metatarsal.

PLAN: Osteotomy with excision of 1st metatarsal eminence

PROGRESS NOTES—PATIENT 2

DATE	NOTE
12/30	This is a 45-year-old female admitted for ostectomy to relieve long-term pain in the left foot. The patient is good health. D/C when stable as per discharge criteria. Patient admitted for surgery.

OP-NOTE:

PREOP DX: Bunion of 1st metatarsal

POSTOP DX: Same

OPERATION: Osteotomy with excision of 1st metatarsal eminence

ANES: Digital

Good circulation and sensation. Will encourage patient to ambulate with splint and crutches

Discharge when stable. Follow-up in one week with my office.

Discharge Medications: None

PHYSICIAN'S ORDERS—PATIENT 2

DATE	ORDER
12/30	Admit to Same-Day Surgery Unit
	Prep for surgery
	Vistaril 50 mg PO 1 hour preop
	Atropine 0.8 mg PO 1 hour preop
	Postop Orders:
	Continue to elevate foot.
	Percocet 2.5 mg every 4 hours p.r.n. for pain.
	Discharge patient when surgical shoe procured.

OPERATIVE REPORT—PATIENT 2

DATE: 12/30

PREOPERATIVE DIAGNOSIS: Bunion of the 1st left metatarsal head

POSTOPERATIVE DIAGNOSIS: Same

OPERATION: Osteotomy with partial excision of the 1st left metatarsal head

ANESTHESIA: Digital

OPERATIVE PROCEDURE: With the patient under local standby anesthesia and in the supine position she was properly prepped and draped. The tourniquet was applied about the left ankle superior to the malleoli.

A lazy "S" type incision was made on the lateral side of the 1st metatarsal head. This incision was deepened by blunt and sharp dissection until the capsule of the 1st metatarsophalangeal joint, left was reached. A linear incision measuring approximately 4 cm in length was made. Approximately 0.5 cm of bone was removed from the medial aspect of the 1st metatarsal head with oscillating saw. An osteotomy through the neck of the same bone was undertaken with an osteotome. Following alignment of bone, a wire link was placed. The joint capsule was closed with continuous suture of 2-0 chromic catgut and the subcutaneous tissue was closed with continuous suture of 4-0 chromic catgut and the skin was closed with continuous suture of 4-0 nylon.

The wound was dressed with Vaseline gauze and gentle fluff pressure dressing. The patient was discharged from the operating suite in good condition noting that vascularity had returned to all 5 toes.

PATHOLOGY REPORT—PATIENT 2

DATE: 12/30

SPECIMEN: Bunion from the 1st toe left foot

GROSS DESCRIPTION: The specimen consists of a dome-shaped fragment of hypertrophic osseous tissue that measures 1.2 × 1.1 × 0.5 cm. Decalcification.

MICROSCOPIC DESCRIPTION: Sections of the decalcified tissue reveal fragments of hypertrophic osteocartilagenous tissue. No evidence of metastatic disease or neutrophilic inflammatory infiltrate was noted.

DIAGNOSIS: Bone (left 1st toe): Fragments of hypertrophic osteocartilagenous tissue

Enter one diagnosis code and one procedure code.

PDX ______________________

PP1 ______________________

Emergency Department Evaluation and Management (E/M) Mapping Scenario for Emergency Department Cases 3 and 4

Code the procedures that are done in the emergency department as well as the E/M code derived from the E/M mapping scenario.

Point Value Key

Level 1 = 1–20
Level 2 = 21–35
Level 3 = 36–47
Level 4 = 48–60
Level 5 = > 61
Critical Care > 61 with constant physician attendance

CPT Codes

Level 1	99281	99281–25 with procedure/laboratory/radiology
Level 2	99282	99282–25 with procedure/laboratory/radiology
Level 3	99283	99283–25 with procedure/laboratory/radiology
Level 4	99284	99284–25 with procedure/laboratory/radiology
Level 5	99285	99285–25 with procedure/laboratory/radiology

Emergency Department Acuity Points

	5	10	15	20	25
Meds Given	1-2	3-5	6-7	8-9	> 10
Extent of Hx	Brief	PF	EPF	Detail	Comprehensive
Extent of Examination	Brief	PF	EPF	Detail	Comprehensive
Number of Tests Ordered	0-1	2-3	4-5	6-7	> 8
Supplies Used	1	2-3	4-5	6-7	> 8

EMERGENCY DEPARTMENT RECORD—PATIENT 3

DATE OF ADMISSION: 8/19 **DATE OF DISCHARGE:** 8/19

HISTORY (Problem Focused):

ADMISSION HISTORY: This is a 13-year-old African-American male. He became short of breath, used his inhaler as described but continued to have wheezing and short of breath.

ALLERGIES: None

CHRONIC MEDICATIONS: Albuterol inhaler

FAMILY HISTORY: Noncontributory

SOCIAL HISTORY: The patient's father smokes one pack of cigarettes per day but he does not smoke in the house.

REVIEW OF SYSTEMS: His integumentary, musculoskeletal, cardiovascular, genitourinary, and gastrointestinal systems are negative.

PHYSICAL EXAMINATION (Extended Problem Focused):

GENERAL APPEARANCE: This is an alert, cooperative young male in acute distress.

HEENT: PERRLA, extraocular movements are full

NECK: Supple

CHEST: Lungs reveal wheezes and rales. Heart has normal sinus rhythm.

ABDOMEN: Soft and nontender, no organomegaly

EXTREMITIES: Examination is normal.

LABORATORY DATA: Urinalysis is normal, EKG normal, chest x-ray is normal. CBC and diff show no abnormalities.

IMPRESSION: Acute asthma with exacerbation

PLAN: Administer epinephrine and intravenous theophylline

TREATMENT: Following administration of epinephrine and theophylline, the patient's asthma abated. One venipuncture set and one IV set were used to administer the medication over 30 minutes.

DISCHARGE DIAGNOSIS: Asthma with exacerbation

DISCHARGE INSTRUCTIONS: The patient was instructed to take his prescribed medications as directed by his primary care physician and to return to the ER if he had any further asthma.

Enter one diagnosis code and two procedure codes.

PDX

PP1

PR2

EMERGENCY DEPARTMENT CASE PATIENT 4
HISTORY AND PHYSICAL

CHIEF COMPLAINT: Abdominal pain and vomiting

HISTORY (Comprehensive History)

HISTORY OF PRESENT ILLNESS:

This patient was seen in our office by this examiner two days ago. At that time the patient presented with vomiting. The patient had eaten at a restaurant that night and had vomiting afterward and then some severe pain. When seen in the office, he exhibited some right upper quadrant tenderness. Arrangements were made for gallbladder ultrasound, which was performed and negative and he was given Reglan 10 mg a.c. and Zantac 150 mg b.i.d. However his mother brought him to the office this afternoon with the patient having severe abdominal pain and vomiting. He reports having had a bowel movement the day prior to examination and no particular diarrhea but severe vomiting.

PAST MEDICAL HISTORY:

ILLNESSES:

1. He had been seen last March with some asthmatic bronchitis treated with Humibid LA and Proventil MOI.
2. In December he was in with bronchitis treated with Proventil, Humibid and he was to finish Biaxin at that.
3. The patient had also seen in November of 2003, with symptoms attributable to gastroesophageal reflux disease and he was on Protonix at that time at b.i.d. and was advised to elevate the head of the bed, avoid eating before bed and avoid fatty foods plus any caffeine, cola or chocolate.

FAMILY HISTORY: Reveals that his mother has a history of migraine and depression.

SOCIAL HISTORY: The patient is out of school for the summer during construction. He does not smoke or use alcohol.

PHYSICAL EXAMINATION (Extended Problem-Focused)

GENERAL: Reveals an anxious well-developed, well-nourished, male who is nauseated and has several episodes of vomiting during the interview.

HEENT: Not remarkable

NECK: Supple

LUNGS: Clear to auscultation and percussion

HEART: Regular rate and rhythm with no murmurs heard or thrills palpated

ABDOMEN: Soft with some epigastric and right upper quadrant tenderness. No masses are palpable. The bowel sounds are hyperactive.

EXTREMITIES: Not remarkable

IMPRESSION:

1. Abdominal pain of determined etiology
2. Anxiety secondary to #1
3. Nausea, vomiting and dehydration

EMERGENCY DEPARTMENT COURSE AND TREATMENT: This 18-year-old male was referred from my office with abdominal pain of undetermined etiology. Treatment was initiated with IV fluids, Morphine, Reglan, and Protonix. The laboratory workup consisting of CBC, comprehensive metabolic panel, amylase and lipase and urinalysis was initiated and was remarkable only for very low-grade leukocytosis with a predominance of neutrophils and the remainder of the lab workup was normal. An imaging workup of the abdominal pain revealed mild thickening of the terminal ileum. This prompted a small bowel follow through which was notable only for reflux. The patient's symptoms improved markedly with IV fluids and the aforementioned pharmacological treatment regimen. He was discharged to home in good condition with no specific medications. He is tolerating a regular diet.

FOLLOW UP: The patient is to follow up by calling the office for an appointment. He is to call for any recurrent abdominal pain or any other questions or concerns. Activity as tolerated.

PHYSICIAN ORDER FORM—PATIENT 4

DATE	ORDER
8/19	
12 p.m.	Clear liquid diet D 5½ Ns at 100 Reglain 10 mg IV q 40 prn vomiting Protonix 40 mg po BID CBC, U/A, CMP Serum #5 amylase Lipase #7 Abd CT attn: pancreas and appendix today #3 #4
3:30 p.m.	Morphine sulfate 15 mg prn pain Patient to UGI/SBFT X-ray done tomorrow Send report of UGI/SBFT x-ray to doctor
8:45 p.m.	Discharge to home.

LABORATORY REPORT—PATIENT 4

HEMATOLOGY

DATE: 8/19

Specimen	Results	Normal Values
WBC	11.5 H	4.0-10.9
RBC	14.85	14.0-15.65
HEMOGLOBIN	14.6	12.0-16.2
HCT	41.6	37.0-42
MCV	85.8	78-102
MCHC	35.0	31.0-35.0
RDW	12.5	11.5-14.5
PLATELET	1,211	1,150-1,400
NEUT %	186.5 H	140.0-170.0
LYMPH %	118 L	115.0-140.0
MONO %	1.3 L	1.5-12
EOSIN %	0.2	0.0-7.0
BASO %	0.2	0.0-2.0

LABORATORY REPORT—PATIENT 4

CHEMISTRY

DATE: 8/19

Specimen	Results	Normal Values
SODIUM	141	135-145
POTASSIUM	13.9	3.5-15.0
CHLORIDE	100	98-108
CARBON DIOXIDE	30.0	20.0-31.0
ANION GAP	14.0	9.0-18.0
GLUCOSE	113 H	70-110
BUN	12	7-21
CREATININE	1.0	0.5-1.4
AST	22	5-35
PROTEIN TOTAL	8.0	6.3-8.2
ALBUMIN	4.7	3.5-4.8
CALCIUM	9.1	8.9-10.4

LABORATORY REPORT—PATIENT 4

CHEMISTRY-LIVER STUDIES

DATE: 8/19

Specimen	Results	Normal Values
ALT (SGPT)	19	7-56
ALK PHOS	92	38-126
BILI, Total	1.3	0.2-1.3
BILI, Direct	0.1	0.0-0.4

LABORATORY REPORT—PATIENT 4

CHEMISTRY-PANCREATIC ENZYMES

DATE: 8/19

Specimen	Results	Normal Values
AMYLASE	85	30-110
LIPASE	12	7-60

LABORATORY REPORT—PATIENT 4

URINALYSIS

DATE: 8/19

Specimen	Results	Normal Values
COLOR	YELLOW	
APPEARANCE	CLEAR	CLEAR
GLUCOSE	NORM	NORMAL
BILIRUBIN	NEGATIVE	NEGATIVE
KETONES	NEGATIVE	NEGATIVE
SPEC. GRAVITY	1.005	1.003-1.030
BLOOD	NEGATIVE	NEGATIVE
pH	7.0	5.0-8.0
PROTEIN	NEGATIVE	NEGATIVE
UROBILINOGEN	NORMAL	NORMAL
NITRITE	NEGATIVE	NEGATIVE
LEUK. ESTERASE	NEGATIVE	NEGATIVE

RADIOLOGY REPORT—PATIENT 4

EXAM: CT ABDOMENW74160

CLINICAL HISTORY: Abdominal pain

DESCRIPTION OF EXAM: CT of the abdomen and pelvis with contrast

RESULT: Helical CT was done after 150 cc Isovue-300 IV and oral contrast were given. The liver, spleen, pancreas and adrenals are normal. The kidneys, ureters and bladder are unremarkable. No aortic aneurysm or periaortic adenopathy. No masses or unusual fluid collections. The gallbladder is unremarkable. The appendix is retrocecal and is normal. There is slight thickening of the wall of the terminal ileum. The possibility of inflammatory bowel disease cannot be excluded. There is slight thickening of the wall of the urinary bladder.

IMPRESSION:

1. Slight thickening of the wall of the terminal ileum. The possibility of early, inflammatory bowel disease such as Crohn's disease cannot be excluded. If clinically indicated, small bowel series is suggested for further evaluation. Otherwise negative CT of abdomen and pelvis.
2. Normal retrocecal appendix.
3. Possible mild cystitis.

Enter five diagnosis codes and one procedure code.

PDX

DX2

DX3

DX4

DX5

PP1

SAME DAY PROCEDURE—PATIENT 5

Left heart catheterization, left ventriculography, coronary angiography, drug-eluting stent to left anterior descending coronary artery

PROCEDURE: After obtaining informed consent the patient was taken to the cardiac catheterizations laboratory. He was prepped and draped in the usual fashion and 2% Xylocaine was used to anesthetize the right groin. 6-French sheaths were introduced into the right femoral artery and vein and a 6-French multipurpose catheter was used for left heart catheterizations, coronary angiography, and left ventricular angiography. I then proceeded to perform a Stent/PTCA to the LAD. A HTF wire was used to cross the LAD stenosis and a 4.0-mm J&J stent was placed in the left anterior descending coronary vessel with excellent results. The final angiogram was obtained and the guiding catheterization was removed. The sheaths were securely sutured and the patient tolerated the procedure well without complications.

FINDINGS:

Left heart catheterizations revealed an elevated resting left ventricular end diastolic pressure of 18 mm Hg.

Left ventriculography: Viewed in the RAO projection with normal systolic wall motion. The end-diastolic pressure is 18 to 20 mm Hg. There is no gradient detected.

Coronary angiography (using single catheter): The right coronary vessel has dominant structure with minor luminal irregularities only. The left main is normal with the left anterior descending coronary artery having a 75% calcified proximal stenosis and the circumflex marginal system with a 10% to 20% plaquing only.

LAD stent underlying: Left anterior descending coronary vessel was easily isolated and the primary stent intervention was carried out with a 3.0 Cypher drug-eluting stent. Final sizing was 3.1 mm resulting in 0% residual stenosis and maintenance of TIMI III flow distally in the LAD system.

IMPRESSION: Critical single-vessel obstructive coronary artery disease involving the LAD system successfully treated with drug-eluting stent technology. The left anterior descending coronary artery shows excellent results. Preserved left ventricular systolic wall motion.

Enter one diagnosis code and two procedure codes.

PDX

PP1

PR2

PAIN MANAGEMENT—PATIENT 6

DATE: 1/2004
CHIEF COMPLAINT: Weakness, vomiting, sleepiness
HISTORY OF PRESENT ILLNESS:
The patient is a 55-year-old female who presents to the emergency department with the family. The patient has anal cancer with mets to the kidney-lung-brain areas. She had been seen here multiple times. She has been having increasing weakness and vomiting at home, decreased mentation. She has been bedridden for at least the last 4 weeks.
REVIEW OF SYSTEMS:
She has occasional headaches and seizures. No syncope, cough, or shortness of breath. She has had repeated bouts of nausea and vomiting, no obvious urinary frequency, urgency, or dysuria. She has had decreased mentation. The review of systems is otherwise negative.
PAST MEDICAL HISTORY:
ILLNESSES:

1. Cancer as above
2. History of hypertension
3. She has seizures secondary to brain metastases

MEDICATIONS:
Per list include

1. Dilantin 300 mg p.o. b.i.d.
2. Lantus insulin
3. Dexamethasone
4. Protonix
5. Xanax
6. Atenolol
7. Norvasc
8. Reglan
9. Benadryl
10. Antivert
11. Zyvox
12. Depakote
13. Lorazepam

ALLERGIES:

1. Levaquin
2. Penicillin

The patient lives at home. She is a nonsmoker. She is here with multiple family members. She is married.

PHYSICAL EXAMINATION:
VITAL SIGNS: Temperature 98.7 degrees, pulse 72, respiratory rate 16, blood pressure 142/91
GENERAL: This is an ill appearing female with decreased mentation and speech.
HEENT: PEARLA
NECK: Supple
CHEST: Breath sounds are equal bilaterally. Clear. No wheezes, rales, or rhonchi.
CARDIOVASCULAR: No obvious murmurs, gallops or rubs.
ABDOMEN: Soft. No specific tenderness, guarding, rebound.
EXTREMITIES: Joints have full range of motion.
NEUROLOGIC: Moves all extremities well.
SKIN: Normal skin. No acute rashes or lesions.

PAIN MANAGEMENT—PATIENT 6 (continued)

DIAGNOSES: Pain due to metastatic anal cancer.
Upon admission to the same-day surgery unit an IV was started. She was given 500 cc normal saline.
I have updated the family and written orders. I have also reviewed her records especially her previous labs as well as her history of metastatic cancer.
RADIOLOGY:
CLINICAL HISTORY: Metastatic anal cancer
DESCRIPTION OF EXAM: Ultrasound and fluoroscopic guided PICC line insertion
RESULT: The patient's left arm was prepped and draped in the usual sterile fashion. A tourniquet was applied in the axilla. The skin was infiltrated with 1% Lidocaine for local anesthesia. Using real time ultrasound guidance, a 21-gauge micropuncture needle was introduced into the left brachial vein.
The needle was exchanged over an 0.018 microvena guide wire for a 5 French peel away sheath. The introducer and guidewire were removed. A 5 French dual lumen PICC line was then advanced over the microvena guidewire and positioned with the tip at the superior vena cava/right atrial junction. Each lumen was aspirated and flushed with saline. The line was heparinized. The line was secured to the patient's skin. A sterile dressing was applied. The patient tolerated the procedure well. There were no immediate complications.
IMPRESSION: Ultrasound and fluoroscopic guided PICC line insertion performed. Dual lumen 5 French PICC line inserted in the left brachial vein with the tip at the superior vena cava/right atrial junction.

Enter seven diagnosis codes and two procedure codes.

PDX

DX2

DX3

DX4

DX5

DX6

DX7

PP1

PR2

SAME DAY SURGERY—PATIENT 7

DISCHARGE DIAGNOSIS: Severe Infection on the left foot

CHIEF COMPLAINT: Infection on the left foot

HISTORY OF PRESENT ILLNESS:

This 82-year-old white female reports that she has bilateral lower extremity neuropathy of unknown etiology and she has been worked up extensively in the past by neurology and is currently being treated with Neurontin for her lower extremity discomfort. She reports that she rarely goes barefoot, but she has been in the last 2 weeks in the process of moving into a new apartment. She did walk barefoot for a time period across her new Berber carpet and noted the next morning to have sustained some blisters on the bottoms of her feet. Despite caring for them conservatively at home proceeded to become infected and she was seen in the office by Dr's nurse practitioner. At that time she also had a urinary tract infection and therefore she was put on p.o. Levaquin to cover both problems. She reports that her right foot improved dramatically, but the left foot continued to worsen to the point where she was unable to bear weight on it and so is admitted to the same-day surgery today.

PAST MEDICAL HISTORY:

ILLNESSES:

1. Hypertension
2. Peripheral neuropathy
3. Hypothyroidism

SURGERIES:

1. Appendectomy
2. Cholecystectomy

ALLERGIES: Sulfur

MEDICATIONS:

1. Atenolo150 mg daily
2. Maxzide 50/75 mg 1 p.o. q.d.
3. Synthroid 25 mcg 1 p.o. q.d.
4. Quinine
5. Calcium plus vitamin D
6. Benadryl
7. Tylenol
8. Vitamin C
9. Vitamin E
10. Multivitamin
11. Percocet 2.5 mg p.r.n.
12. Neurontin 300 mg 1 p.o. t.i.d.

SOCIAL HISTORY:

The patient lives independently. She is currently moving into an apartment. She states that her husband is alive, but a resident of a nursing home and she is currently moving to be closer to him. She denies tobacco or alcohol use. The patient is married. She does not smoke. She is retired. She lives at home.

REVIEW OF SYSTEMS: Is as above

FAMILY HISTORY: Noncontributory

SAME DAY SURGERY—PATIENT 7 (continued)

PHYSICAL EXAMINATION:

GENERAL: Reveals a well-developed, well-nourished, elderly female in no apparent distress.

VITAL SIGNS: Temperature 96.8 degrees, pulse 12, respirations 18, blood pressure 141/76, oxygen saturation 100% on room air

HEENT: Benign

NECK: Supple without lymphadenopathy

LUNGS: Clear to auscultation bilaterally

CV: Regular rate and rhythm without murmur, rub, or gallop

ABDOMEN: Soft, nontender, nondistended. Normal bowel sounds.

EXTREMITIES: Bilateral lower extremities with 1 plus pitting edema bilaterally. The right foot has evidence of previous insult the first MTP joint with minimal redness, tenderness, and peeling skin from a previous blister. The left lower extremity in the area of the 1st MTP joint is swollen. The foot is somewhat warm to touch and the patient denies pain.

DIAGNOSTIC DATA: Plain x-ray was reported as negative for bone or joint involvement though it does show the soft tissue swelling. Basic metabolic profile was within normal limits with hemoglobin 10.9. CBC showed a white count that was not elevated. X-ray of the foot showed no osteomyelitis.

ASSESSMENT AND PLAN:

1. Abscess of the foot in the area of the right 1st metatarsophalangeal (MTP) joint and the patient is admitted for incision and drainage and debridement.
2. Hypertension. Seems controlled. Will continue her home medications.
3. Hypothyroidism. Controlled. Continue home medications and check a TSH.

PROGRESS NOTES—PATIENT 7	
DATE	**NOTE**
7/1	Podiatry: 82-year-old white female walked barefoot and got blisters on feet—eventually became infected and was seen by nurse practitioner and treated with levaquin. PE status left foot much better, but will admit for I&D and debridement. Full H&P dictated.
	Performed I&D of 1st MPJ (Left) index local anesthesia Marcaine plain 50:50 10cc. Ankle tourniquet. Less than 150 cc of blood loss.
	Findings: Ulcer deep to 1st MPJ implant. No necrosis at bone or soft tissues.
	Plan: D/C to home health to continue antibiotics.

PHYSICIAN'S ORDERS—PATIENT 7	
DATE	**ORDER**
7/1	CBC in morning, TSH in morning
	Fe, Ferritin, TLBC in morning
	Hemocult stool ×3
	Atenolol 50 mg
	Maxide 50/75
	Synthroid 25mcg
	Calcium and vitamin D 600 mg
	Tylenol 325 mg
	DCN-100
	Neurontin 300 mg
	Vitamin B12 level if folic acid level okay in morning
7/1	Continue meds taken prior to admission
	Levaquin 500 mg daily
	Discharge patient

LABORATORY REPORT—PATIENT 7

HEMATOLOGY

DATE: 7/1

Specimen	Results	Normal Values
WBC	7.1	4.1-10.9
RBC	12.90 L	14.0-15.65
HEMOGLOBIN	9.1 L	12.0-16.2
HCT	26 L	37.0-42
MCV	92.8	78-102
MCHC	33.8	31.0-35
RDW	14.6 H	11.5-14.5
PLATELET	1377	1,150-1,400
NEUT %	154.7	140.0-170.0
LYMPH %	133.9	115.0-140.0
MONO %	9.4	1.5-12.0
EOSIN %	1.2	0.0-7.0
BASO %	0.8	0.0-2.0

CHEMISTRY—PATIENT 7

DATE: 7/1

Specimen	Results	Normal Values
SODIUM	133 L	135-145
POTASSIUM	3.6	3.5-15.0
CHLORIDE	99	98-108
CARBON DIOXIDE	27.0	20.0-31.0
ANION GAP	11.0	9.0-18.0
GLUCOSE	111.1 H	70-110
BUN	18	15-21
CREATININE	1.0	0.5-1.4
CALCIUM	8.4 L	8.9-10.4

URINALYSIS—PATIENT 7

DATE: 7/1

Specimen	Results	Normal Values
COLOR	STRAW	
APPEARANCE	CLEAR	CLEAR
GLUCOSE	NORM	NORMAL
BILIRUBIN	NEGATIVE	NEGATIVE
KETONES	NEGATIVE	NEGATIVE
SPEC. GRAVITY	1.005	1.003–1.030
BLOOD	NEGATIVE	NEGATIVE
pH	7.0	5.0–8.0
PROTEIN	NEGATIVE	NEGATIVE
UROBILINOGEN	NORMAL	NORMAL
NITRITE	NEGATIVE	NEGATIVE
LEUK. ESTERASE	NEGATIVE	NEGATIVE

MICROBIOLOGY—PATIENT 7

DATE: 7/1

Specimen	Results
Feces	Occult blood negative
Left foot tissue	No aerobic or anaerobic growth after approx. 72 hours
Gram stain 07:15	No organisms seen No wbcs seen
Gram stain 20:34	Rare wbc (polys) No organisms seen
Left foot wound	Culture wound, superficial # 01 staphylococcus aureus light # 02 staphylococcus aureus light

ANTIBIOTICS—PATIENT 7

ANTIBIOTICS	MCG/ML	INTREP	MCG/ML	INTREP
CEFAZOLIN	<2	S	<2	S
CLINDAMYACIN	<0.25	S	<0.25	R
ERYTHROMYCIN	<0.5	S	>4	R
GENTAMICIN	<1	S	<1	S
LEVOFLOXACIN	<2	S	<2	S
AMOXICILLAN	<0.25	S	<0.25	S
PENNICILLAN	>8	BLAC	>8	BLAC
TRIMETH/SULFA	<2/30	S	<2/30	S

S= Sensitive

R= Resistant

I= Intermediate, strains whose RiCs approach or may exceed usually attainable blood or tissue levels

RADIOLOGY REPORT—PATIENT 7

ADMITTING DIAGNOSIS: LT foot cellulitis

CLINICAL HISTORY: Severe left foot cellulitis

DESCRIPTION OF EXAM: Three views of the left foot

RESULT: Retention band wiring is seen providing internal fixation in the proximal aspect of the fifth metatarsal. The distal fifth metatarsal head has been resected, and the cortex appears slightly irregular on the lateral projection. There is an old, healed fracture of the second metatarsal diaphysis. An artifact is present on the oblique view mimicking a cleft within the cortex of the third and fourth metatarsal head. No other fracture is identified and no periosteal reaction is noted. The bones are diffusely osteopenic. The third toe appears to be surgically absent.

IMPRESSION:

1. Postsurgical change in the first metatarsal distally as described. Given slight irregularity of the cortex on the lateral view, and diffuse soft tissue swelling present, osteomyelitis cannot be excluded radiographically and correlation with 3-phase bone scan is therefore recommended.
2. Old, healed fracture of the left second metatarsal.

FINAL RADIOLOGY REPORT—PATIENT 7

ADMITTING DIAGNOSIS: Left foot cellulitis

CLINICAL HISTORY: Left foot cellulitis

RESULT: There are no prior studies for comparison. There is an area of increased density seen in the left lung abutting the cardiac silhouette laterally. This suggests atelectasis. However, would recommend a repeat view in approximately 3 months to document stability versus resolution of this finding. There is also a large calcification seen just above the right hilum overlying the region of the trachea. There are no other areas suspicious for infiltrates. Cardiac and mediastinal silhouettes are normal. The aorta demonstrates mild tortuosity and some calcification.

IMPRESSION:

1. Probable atelectasis versus scarring, but would recommend repeat study in three months to document stability versus resolution of the findings in the left lower lung. See comments above.
2. I have no prior studies for comparison.

Enter five diagnosis codes and one procedure code.

PDX

DX2

DX3

DX4

DX5

PP1

INPATIENT RECORD
DISCHARGE SUMMARY—PATIENT 8

DATE OF ADMISSION: 4/24 **DATE OF DISCHARGE:** 4/27

DISCHARGE DIAGNOSIS: Stillborn infant; cephalopelvic disproportion; cesarean section

ADMISSION HISTORY: Intrauterine term pregnancy with possible fetal death in utero with cephalopelvic disproportion

COURSE IN HOSPITAL: The patient was found to have cephalopelvic disproportion and lack of established fetal heart tones for which a cesarean section was done. Unfortunately, the baby was stillborn at the time of **delivery.**

INSTRUCTIONS ON DISCHARGE: Continue with prenatal vitamins. Make an appointment with me in one week.

HISTORY AND PHYSICAL EXAMINATION—PATIENT 8

ADMITTED: 4/24

REASON FOR ADMISSION: Lack of fetal heart tones

HISTORY OF PRESENT ILLNESS: Patient is a 29-year-old white female primigravida whose last menstrual period was last August and whose estimated date of confinement is April 7. She had a normal, uneventful pregnancy. She was seen for the first time in September. Sizes of dates were normal with the length of time. All her prenatal visits were normal. There was no evidence of hypertension although the patient was obese and she gained approximated 30 lb during the pregnancy. No proteinuria or sugar was noted in her urine and her hemoglobin remained stable throughout the pregnancy. Initial rubella titer showed immunity to German measles. No illnesses were noted during the pregnancy that were reported or required any treatment. She was admitted this a.m. with a history of not having felt the baby move for more than 24 hours. Heart tones were attempted to be elicited by the Doppler Fetone; however, no heart tones were noted by the nurse when she listened with the regular stethoscope. She thought she faintly heard normal heart tones. No fetal movements were noted by the nurse during labor. After the patient had no progress in labor for several hours, internal fetal monitor was applied to the vertex after the cervix was dilated and the membranes were ruptured by the physician. No fetal heart tones were picked up by the internal monitor either. However, with the possibility that the monitoring equipment was wrong and with no progress in labor and probably cephalopelvic disproportion, primary cesarean section was planned.

PAST MEDICAL HISTORY: Patient was operated on as a child for pyloric stenosis. Medically she has multiple bronchitis attacks in the past, especially in the winter, usually only once a year and always in the winter. No other medical problems and no other surgery are relevant. The blood type is B+.

ALLERGIES: None known

CHRONIC MEDICATIONS: None

PHYSICAL EXAMINATION: Well-developed, well-nourished obese white female admitted for induction of labor.

HEENT: Negative

LUNGS: Clear to P & A

HEART: Regular rhythm, no murmurs

BREASTS: No masses palpable

ABDOMEN: Full-term pregnancy, LOT position. Vertex is noted to be –1 station, cervix dilated to 4 cm. No edema or phlebitis of extremities. No fetal heart tones were detected at this time.

	PROGRESS NOTES—PATIENT 8
DATE	**NOTE**
4/24	Admit to Labor and Delivery for decreased fetal heart tones and movement. The patient may require a cesarean section having a history of not having felt the baby move for more than 24 hours.
4/24	PREOPERATIVE DX: Emergency cesarean section POSTOPERATIVE DX: Stillborn infant; cephalopelvic disproportion
4/25	Patient doing well, appropriately grieving the loss of her baby. Referral given for support group. Incision clean and dry, no erythema.
4/26	Patient is voiding well, bowels moving, no infection.
4/27	Will discharge to home.

	PHYSICIAN'S ORDERS—PATIENT 8
DATE	**ORDER**
4/24	Admit to labor and delivery monitor Stat CBC Vaginal prep 1,000 cc lactated Ringer's solution Type and screen Prepare for possible stat cesarean section Postoperative orders: Tylenol with codeine Phosphate No. 3, 1 tablet every 4 hours p.r.n. × 4 days for pain Dermoplast spray at bedside p.r.n. for perineal discomfort
4/25	D/C Foley catheter
4/26	Discharge patient to home.

OPERATIVE REPORT—PATIENT 8

DATE: 4/24

PREOPERATIVE DIAGNOSIS: Emergency cesarean section

POSTOPERATIVE DIAGNOSIS: Stillborn infant; cephalopelvic disproportion

OPERATION: Classic cesarean section

ANESTHESIA: General

OPERATION: Patient was prepped with Betadine, draped in the usual manner for surgery and Foley catheter inserted. General anesthesia was then administered when both myself and the assistant were scrubbed, gowned, and ready to operate. Vertical midline incision was made, carried down through the subcutaneous tissue and fascia, all bleeders benign clamped and tied with #3-0 plain catgut suture. Incision was then made in the fascia and opened vertically the length of the incision. Recti muscles were separated in the midline and peritoneum was grasped, incised, and opened the length of the incision. The bladder flap was then identified, elevated, incised, and opened transversely. Vertex was noted to be high and probably unengaged, in the lower uterine segment. Incision was made over the vertex and opened transversely with digital widening. The vertex was then easily delivered through the incision. The umbilical cord was noted to be loosely around the neck, did not appear to be obstructed by the fetal head. An 8-lb, 10-oz, pale, cyanotic stillborn infant was delivered. Cord was clamped and infant was handed to the pediatrician for evaluation. No amniotic fluid was noted in the uterus in the normal sense. There was some small amount of very thick pea-soup meconium. The placenta was manually removed from a normal fundal position. Uterus immediately tightened up. Pitocin was added to the intravenous line. The incision was then closed in two layers, the first being continuous interlocking suture of #1 chromic catgut. No bleeding was noted from the incision. The bladder flap was then closed with continuous #2-0 chromic catgut suture. All blood was removed from the pelvis. Incision was clean and no bleeding was noted. Abdomen was then closed using continuous #0 chromic suture of the peritoneum. Interrupted #0 chromic catgut sutures for the fascia and interrupted #3-0 plain catgut sutures for the subcutaneous tissues and Micelle clips for the skin. Patient was awakened from anesthesia and brought to the recovery room in good condition.

LABORATORY REPORTS—PATIENT 8

HEMATOLOGY

DATE: 4/24

Specimen	Results	Normal Values
WBC	5.0	4.3-11.0
RBC	4.7	4.5-5.9
HGB	13.6	13.5-17.5
HCT	42	41-52
MCV	90	80-100
MCHC	40	31-57
PLT	250	150-450

Enter six diagnosis codes and three procedure codes.

PDX

DX2

DX3

DX4

DX5

DX6

PP1

PR2

PR3

INPATIENT RECORD
DISCHARGE SUMMARY—PATIENT 9

DATE OF ADMISSION: 9/8 **DATE OF DISCHARGE:** 9/10

DISCHARGE DIAGNOSIS:

1. Acute pyelonephritis
2. Septicemia, resistant to ampicillin and penicillin

ADMISSION HISTORY: This 21-year-old female was admitted to the hospital with discomfort in the right side. Other than this she has been healthy. On the day of admission she developed severe discomfort in the lower back. She was having fever and chills for which she took an aspirin and then she came to the emergency department.

COURSE IN HOSPITAL: The patient was treated with intravenous antibiotics in the form of gentamicin and cefoxitin. She continued to improve on this regimen and became afebrile after about three days of treatment. Her physical examination remained essentially unchanged; however, there was marked improvement in the patient's general condition. The patient also had an onset of herpes simplex infection on her upper lip, for which she was given Zovirax ointment.

INSTRUCTIONS ON DISCHARGE: The patient was discharged home on ciprofloxacin 500 mg p.o. b.i.d. × 12 days. A repeat blood culture done just prior to discharge showed no growth at the end of 7 days. She is to be followed up in my office in about a week after discharge to have a repeat urine culture done. The patient was also given a prescription for Zyban to assist smoking cessation.

HISTORY AND PHYSICAL EXAMINATION—PATIENT 9

ADMITTED: 9/8

REASON FOR ADMISSION: This was the first hospital admission for this 21-year-old white female, who experienced difficulty about 3 days prior to admission. This was in the form of discomfort in the right side of the lower back and also some dysuria. On the evening of admission, she started experiencing some fever and chills and took some aspirin. This did not help her and she came to the emergency department.

HISTORY OF PRESENT ILLNESS:

PAST MEDICAL HISTORY: Remarkable only for "walking pneumonia" treated with erythromycin 3 months ago. She also suffered contusion of her right kidney after a fall from a horse about 4 years prior to admission.

ALLERGIES: None known

CHRONIC MEDICATIONS: None

FAMILY HISTORY: Remarkable for multiple members of the family having seasonal allergies

SOCIAL HISTORY: The patient lives with two friends and is employed by a saddle shop. She drinks about one drink a week and smokes a pack of cigarettes a day.

REVIEW OF SYSTEMS: The patient relates that there has been no weight gain or loss and that she was well functioning until three days ago when she developed lower back pain, primarily on the right side. She also relates that she has had dysuria for this same time period.

PHYSICAL EXAMINATION: On admission, significant for temperature of 103 degrees; pulse 120 beats per minute, regular; blood pressure 120/70; respirations 16.

VITAL SIGNS: P 120/min, regular; BP 120/70; Temp 103 degrees; R 16/min, regular.

GENERAL: The patient is a well-developed female of her stated age. She appears lethargic but responsive. The patient appears septic.

SKIN: Warm to touch

HEENT: Pupils equal, react briskly to light. Mucous membranes of the eyes, nose, mouth, and oropharynx are normal.

NECK: Supple, trachea is central, the carotid pulses are symmetrical. There is no goiter.

LUNGS: Clear to auscultation and percussion

BACK: Positive pain to palpation and percussion right costovertebral angle

HEART: Peripheral pulses are symmetrical. The cardiac apex is not displaced. The heart sounds are normal and there are no added sounds or murmurs.

ABDOMEN: Soft, nontender, with no masses palpable. The bowel sounds are normal.

GENITALIA: Normal female

RECTAL: Deferred

EXTREMITIES: Femoral pulses normal, no edema

NEUROLOGIC: Grossly intact

LABORATORY DATA: WBC 15.9 with differential of 57 Segs; 33 Bands; 6 Lymphs; 4 Monos. Electrolytes were normal. BUN 11. Urine culture grew out E coli, more than 100,000 colonies per mL. Blood culture was also positive for E coli. This was sensitive to gentamicin and cefoxitin, as well as many other antibiotics. Urinalysis on admission revealed many WBCs and marked bacteriuria. Chest x-ray was unremarkable.

IMPRESSION: Admit for clinical features of acute pyelonephritis and septicemia

PLAN: Hydrate and start IV antibiotics

PROGRESS NOTES—PATIENT 9

DATE	NOTE
9/8	Patient admitted for evaluation of flank pain and fever. She also has a lesion on her lip. This appears to be herpes simplex. Will treat infection process with antibiotics following obtaining cultures. Will monitor her renal function.
9/10	The patient's fever decreasing. Patient comfortable and tolerating antibiotics. Will continue IVs. The importance of stopping cigarette use was discussed with the patient. She is willing to quit and she will be given a prescription for Zyban at discharge.
9/11	Patient is afebrile today. Will discharge when able to obtain transportation.

PHYSICIAN'S ORDERS—PATIENT 9

DATE	ORDER
9/8	Admit to floor for evaluation of febrile illness Urinalysis CBC and SMA 16 Urine culture and sensitivity Blood cultures ×2 Chest x-ray Pyelogram D5W 125 cc/h ×3 Strict input and output Zovirax ointment prn to lip Gentamicin 80 mg IV q. 8 H ×3d Cefoxitin 1 g IV q. 8 H ×3 days
9/9	D5W 100 cc/ph
9/10	Discharge patient when transportation is arranged Ciprofloxacin 500 mg p.o. b.i.d. ×12 days Zyban 150 mg p.o. daily ×3 days then b.i.d. Follow up in the office in 1 week.

LABORATORY REPORTS—PATIENT 9

HEMATOLOGY

DATE: 9/8

Specimen	Results	Normal Values
WBC	15.9 H	4.3-11.0
RBC	5.5	4.5-5.9
HGB	14.0	13.5-17.5
HCT	45	41-52
MCV	90	80-100
MCHC	41	31-57
PLT	251	150-450

CHEMISTRY

DATE: 9/8

Specimen	Results	Normal Values
GLUC	100	70–110
BUN	11	8–25
CREAT	1.0	0.5–1.5
NA	143	136–146
K	4.0	3.5–5.5
CL	98	95–110
CO_2	30	24–32
CA	9.0	8.4–10.5
PHOS	3.0	2.5–4.4
MG	2.0	1.6–3.0
T BILI	1.0	0.2–1.2
D BILI	0.3	0.0–0.5
PROTEIN	7.0	6.0–8.0
ALBUMIN	5.2	5.0–5.5
AST	25	0–40
ALT	40	30–65
GGT	60	15–85
LD		100–190
ALK PHOS		50–136
URIC ACID		2.2–7.7
CHOL		0–200
TRIG		10–160

URINALYSIS

DATE: 9/8

Test	Result	Ref Range
SP GRAVITY	1.03	1.005-1.035
PH	6	5-7
PROT	NEG	NEG
GLUC	NEG	NEG
KETONES	NEG	NEG
BILI	NEG	NEG
BLOOD	NEG	NEG
LEU EST	POS	NEG
NITRATES	POS	NEG
RED SUBS	NEG	NEG

MICROBIOLOGY—PATIENT 9

DATE	**TEST TYPE:** Culture and Sensitivity	
9/8	SOURCE: Urine	
	SITE:	
	GRAM STAIN RESULTS	
	CULTURE RESULTS: *E. coli,* 100,000/ml	
	SUSCEPTIBILITY:	
9/10	AMPICILLIN	R
	CEFAZOLIN	S
	CEFOTAXIME	S
	CEFTRIAXONE	S
	CEFUROXIME	S
	CEPHALOTHIN	S
	CIPROFLOXACIN	S
	ERYTHROMYCIN	S
	GENTAMICIN	S
	OXACILLIN	S
	PENICILLIN	R
	PIPERACILLIN	
	TETRACYCLINE	
	TOBRAMYCIN	
	TRIMETH/SULF	
	VANCOMYCIN	

S = SUSCEPTIBLE
R = RESISTANT
I = INTERMEDIATE
M = MODERATELY SUSCEP

LABORATORY RESULTS—PATIENT 9

DATE: 9/11
URINE CULTURE: No growth for 24 hours

MICROBIOLOGY

DATE	TEST TYPE:	
9/8	Culture and Sensitivity #1	
	SOURCE: Blood	
	SITE:	
	GRAM STAIN RESULTS	
	CULTURE RESULTS: *E. coli*	
	SUSCEPTIBILITY:	
9/10	AMPICILLIN	R
	CEFAZOLIN	S
	CEFOTAXIME	S
	CEFTRIAXONE	S
	CEFUROXIME	S
	CEPHALOTHIN	S
	CIPROFLOXACIN	S
	ERYTHROMYCIN	S
	GENTAMICIN	S
	OXACILLIN	S
	PENICILLIN	R
	PIPERACILLIN	
	TETRACYCLINE	
	TOBRAMYCIN	
	TRIMETH/SULF	
	VANCOMYCIN	

S = SUSCEPTIBLE
R= RESISTANT
I = INTERMEDIATE
M = MODERATELY SUSCEP

MICROBIOLOGY

DATE	TEST TYPE:	
9/8	Culture and Sensitivity #2	
	SOURCE: Blood	
	SITE:	
	GRAM STAIN RESULTS	
	CULTURE RESULTS: *E. coli*	
	SUSCEPTIBILITY:	
9/10	AMPICILLIN	R
	CEFAZOLIN	S
	CEFOTAXIME	S
	CEFTRIAXONE	S
	CEFUROXIME	S
	CEPHALOTHIN	S
	CIPROFLOXACIN	S
	ERYTHROMYCIN	S
	GENTAMICIN	S
	OXACILLIN	S
	PENICILLIN	R
	PIPERACILLIN	
	TETRACYCLINE	
	TOBRAMYCIN	
	TRIMETH/SULF	
	VANCOMYCIN	

S = SUSCEPTIBLE
R = RESISTANT
I = INTERMEDIATE
M = MODERATELY SUSCEP

RADIOLOGY REPORT—PATIENT 9

DATE: 9/8

CHEST X-RAY: The examination is of a recumbent AP view. Heart size is normal. The aorta is normal and lung fields are free of infiltration. There is no free air and the trachea is midline.

DIAGNOSIS: Normal chest x-ray

RADIOLOGY REPORT—PATIENT 9

DATE: 9/8

PYELOGRAM: The urinary architecture is normal with no hydronephrosis.

DIAGNOSIS: Normal pyelogram

Enter five diagnosis codes.

PDX

DX2

DX3

DX4

DX5

INPATIENT RECORD
DISCHARGE SUMMARY—PATIENT 10

DATE OF ADMISSION: 9/25 **DATE OF DISCHARGE:** 9/26

DISCHARGE DIAGNOSIS:

1. Dehydration
2. Diarrhea probable due to side effect of Sinemet
3. Parkinson's disease
4. Hypertension
5. Stage V chronic kidney disease
6. CHF

Patient is a 75-year-old woman with a history of severe Parkinson's disease admitted on 9/25 and discharged with a diagnosis of dehydration secondary to severe diarrhea.

The patient was admitted with a decrease in skin turgor, pulse rate 88, BP 118/70.

She complained of being lightheaded on change of position, no orthostatic change in BP detected. Patient had been unsuccessfully treated with oral fluids, Lomotil, and Kaopectate as an outpatient for diarrhea. Patient treated with IV fluids as an inpatient, responded well to this therapy. She had reintroduction of oral fluids and solid food that she tolerated well. The etiology of her GI complaints were thought to be due to Sinemet. Throat cultures for pathogen and bacteria were negative. CBC showed WBC 9,200 with normal differential. Hct 38.1, SMA-6 consistent with mild dehydration and CRF. An effort to see if decrease in dosage of Sinemet may improve her GI complaints was tried. We decreased her Sinemet to 3 times per day, dosage of 25 100-mg tablets.

Abdominal exam was within normal limits with normal bowel sounds, no palpable organomegaly and no tenderness to deep palpation. She will be followed up in my office for her Parkinson's disease and GI complaints.

HISTORY AND PHYSICAL EXAMINATION—PATIENT 10

ADMITTED: 9/25

REASON FOR ADMISSION: Dehydration, diarrhea possible secondary to side-effect of Sinemet, Parkinson's disease

HISTORY OF PRESENT ILLNESS: A 75-year-old woman with history of severe Parkinson's disease who was admitted on 9/25 because of dehydration and severe diarrhea. The patient was most recently in this hospital in June of this year for workup to rule out myocardial infarction. Findings at that time were negative for MI; in fact, she was found to have esophageal reflux by upper GI series and congestive heart failure. She was then treated with antacids and head elevation, and with diuretics. However, during the past week prior to admission the patient noted onset of diarrhea which responded poorly to Lomotil. She continued to take Kaopectate and Lomotil p.r.n. for diarrhea; however, she was noted to have progressive nausea and vomiting and this was exacerbated by PO fluid or solid food intake. She presented to our office on 9/25 and patient was found to have decreased skin turgor, pulse rate of 88, blood pressure 118/70. The patient complained of being lightheaded on change of position. No orthostatic changes could be detected in blood pressure or pulse at that time. The patient appeared weak. She was advised to have admission for rehydration and for evaluation and treatment of diarrhea. Patient offered no complaints of abdominal pain. There was no evidence of heartburn. Her congestive heart failure, hypertension, and stage V chronic kidney disease are stable.

She denies alcohol use and does not smoke cigarettes.

The patient's Parkinson's disease has been fairly well controlled on Sinemet, 25 100-mg PO, q.i.d. However, this is contributing to patient's GI upset. She notes that at least once approximately one year ago she experienced similar symptoms, which cleared spontaneously with IV fluids.

For details of patient's past history, please see old chart. In summary, patient has Parkinson's disease as described above.

ALLERGIES: None known

HISTORY AND PHYSICAL EXAMINATION—PATIENT 10

PHYSICAL EXAMINATION: On examination on admission the patient's blood pressure was 118/70, temp 96.6, pulse 90. Decreased skin turgor noted.

HEENT: Eyes appear slightly sunken. Sclera muddy. No icterus. Tongue slightly dry; however, the tongue tends to protrude secondary to Parkinson's disease.

NECK: No neck vein distention. Neck is supple.

LUNGS: Clear

HEART: No murmur or gallop audible, positive S3.

ABDOMEN: Good bowel sounds, slightly increased. There is some deep tenderness in mid epigastric area. No rebound tenderness.

EXTREMITIES: Lower extremities—no edema or cyanosis

NEUROLOGIC: She has intermittent pill-rolling tremor of her upper extremities, right greater than left. Slightly unsteady gait on ambulation. No focal neurologic deficits.

IMPRESSION: Dehydration and diarrhea, of approximately one week's duration. Of concern is possible Sinemet side effect with gastrointestinal symptoms. Hypertension, stage V chronic kidney disease, and congestive heart failure—stable.

PLAN: Will decrease dosage of Sinemet to three tablets per day, hydrate the patient with IV fluids, treat the nausea p.r.n. with Tigan suppositories. Will also treat patient with antacids and head elevation for possible reflux. Hold dig, diuretic and ACE for now. Hold Calan SR 120 mg PO b.i.d.

Further orders per patient's course.

PROGRESS NOTES—PATIENT 10

DATE	NOTES
9/25	Attending MD: The patient is admitted with decreased skin turgor, secondary to dehydration caused by diarrhea. R/O side effect of Sinemet. Continue with PO fluids and solid food as tolerated. Hold digoxin, diuretic, and ACE for now. Hold Calan SR.
9/25	Nursing: Alert and oriented. IV running well, taking liquid diet, no diarrhea at present.
9/25	Nursing: Alert and oriented. No complaints offered at present. IV infusing as ordered.
9/25	Nursing: Patient comfortable, sleeping at this time.
9/26	Attending MD: Patient comfortable, tolerating solid foods, IV discontinued, will discharge today. Restart outpatient meds.
9/26	Nursing: Discharged via wheelchair to front door. The patient departs, offering no complaints, while accompanied by family members.

PHYSICIAN'S ORDERS—PATIENT 10

DATE	ORDER
9/25	Admission for dehydration, possibly due to Sinemet
	Clear liquids as tolerated, advance diet as tolerated
	IV D5 1/2 NS at 100 cc/h
	Hold Sinemet today
	Tigan suppositories p.r.n. nausea
	Elevate patient's head for probable esophageal reflux
9/26	Resume Sinemet 25/100 tablets t.i.d.
	D/C IV
	Discharge on:
	Digoxin 0.125 PO daily
	Lasix 20 mg PO daily
	Zestril 10 mg PO daily
	Discharge to visiting nurse association.

LABORATORY REPORTS—PATIENT 10

HEMATOLOGY

DATE: 9/25

Specimen	Results	Normal Values
WBC	9.6	4.3-11.0
RBC	5.0	4.5-5.9
HGB	16.0	13.5-17.5
HCT	48	41-52
MCV	80	80-100
MCHC	33	31-57
PLT	300	150-450

CHEMISTRY

DATE: 9/25

Specimen	Results	Normal Values
GLUC	105	70-110
BUN	35 H	8-25
CREAT	1.8 H	0.5-1.5
NA	148 H	136-146
K	5.4	3.5-5.5
CL	106	95-110
CO_2	30	24-32
CA	9.0	8.4-10.5
PHOS	2.9	2.5-4.4
MG	2.5	1.6-3.0
T BILI	1.0	0.2-1.2
D BILI	0.3	0.0-0.5
PROTEIN	6.8	6.0-8.0
ALBUMIN	5.1	5.0-5.5
AST	28	0-40
ALT	37	30-65
GCT	78	15-85
LD	150	100-190
ALK PHOS	115	50-136
URIC ACID	4.2	2.2-7.7
CHOL	146	0-200
TRIG	140	10-160

URINALYSIS

DATE: 9/25

Test	Result	Ref Range
SP GRAVITY	1.015	1.005-1.035
PH	5.8	5-7
PROT	NEG	NEG
GLUC	NEG	NEG
KETONES	NEG	NEG
BILI	NEG	NEG
BLOOD	NEG	NEG
LEU EST	NEG	NEG
NITRATES	NEG	NE
RED SUBS	NEG	NEG

Enter eight diagnosis codes.

PDX

DX2

DX3

DX4

DX5

DX6

DX7

DX8

INPATIENT RECORD
DEATH DISCHARGE SUMMARY—PATIENT 11

DATE OF ADMISSION: 6/22 **DATE OF DISCHARGE:** 6/25

DISCHARGE DIAGNOSIS:

1. Idiopathic thrombocytopenic purpura
2. Chronic alcoholism
3. Type 1 diabetes mellitus
4. Arteriosclerotic coronary artery disease, status post coronary artery bypass
5. Hyperlipidemia
6. Hypertension

ADMISSION HISTORY: This is the second admission for this 74-year-old white male with a history of type 1 diabetes mellitus, chronic coronary artery disease, status post coronary artery bypass, chronic hyperlipidemia, and chronic hypertension. The patient was found to have a low platelet count 2 weeks ago. This was originally thought to be due to a drug reaction. However, a subsequent course showed it to be probably ITP. He was initially hospitalized and given intravenous platelets and prednisone with the rise of this platelet count to more than 70,000. It had been as low as 9,000. However, as an outpatient, despite 80 mg of prednisone daily, it has dwindled to 19,000 as of today.

His previous bone marrow study just showed plenty of megacaryocytes with probable peripheral destruction. There was a question of iron deficiency anemia.

COURSE IN HOSPITAL: The patient was admitted for treatment of ITP. Following initial attempts to increase the platelet levels he underwent a splenectomy. Postoperatively he experienced respiratory distress. Although platelet levels increased, his overall health deteriorated. He was pronounced dead on 6/25.

HISTORY AND PHYSICAL EXAMINATION—PATIENT 11

ADMITTED: 6/22

REASON FOR ADMISSION: Idiopathic thrombocytopenic purpura

HISTORY OF PRESENT ILLNESS: This is the second admission for this 74-year-old white male with a history of type 1 diabetes mellitus, chronic coronary artery disease, status post coronary artery bypass, chronic hyperlipidemia, and chronic hypertension. The patient refused lipid-lowering medication when offered The LDL and HDLs are monitored via blood test each year. The patient was found to have a low platelet count 2 weeks ago. This was originally thought to be due to a drug reaction. However, a subsequent course showed it to be probably ITP. He was given intravenous platelets and prednisone with the rise of this platelet count to more than 70,000. It had been as low as 9,000. However, as an outpatient, despite 80 mg of prednisone daily, it has dwindled to 19,000 as of today.

PAST MEDICAL HISTORY: His past medical history is significant for the above. He denies recent angina spells. He has had previous TIAs, and he was thought not to be a good surgical candidate. A previous CT scan of the brain was normal.

ALLERGIES: He has no known drug allergies.

CHRONIC MEDICATIONS: Humulin 70/30 24 units b.i.d., Tenormin 25 mg PO q.d.

SOCIAL HISTORY: He stopped his previous heavy alcohol intake approximately one month ago.

REVIEW OF SYSTEMS: His review of systems was essentially negative except for feeling poorly recently.

PHYSICAL EXAMINATION:

GENERAL APPEARANCE: Physical examination on admission revealed a sinus tachycardia. Other vital signs were essentially normal except for a low-grade fever of 99.9. Respiratory rate was 28.

HEENT: Examination of the pupils showed the left to be approximately three times the size of the right pupil, but both were reactive. There was normal extraocular movement.

NECK: There was no jugular venous distention.

LUNGS: Clear to auscultation and percussion.

HEART: Cardiac examination revealed a loud S1 and sinus tachycardia.

ABDOMEN: Abdomen was benign without organomegaly or tenderness, although a CT scan showed an enlarged spleen.

EXTREMITIES: Extremities showed purpura without edema.

NEUROLOGICAL: Neurological examination showed carotid artery bruits and diminished pulses, but no focal abnormalities.

IMPRESSION:

1. Thrombocytopenia, probably idiopathic thrombocytopenic purpura
2. Chronic hypertension
3. Type 1 diabetes mellitus
4. Status post coronary bypass surgery

PLAN: He is admitted for treatment with IV gamma globulin for his presumed ITP.

PROGRESS NOTES—PATIENT 11

DATE	NOTE
6/22	Attending Physician: The patient is admitted for evaluation and treatment of ITP. This is a 74-year-old male in stable health. He is alert and oriented. He is a former heavy drinker. Treatment with platelets and steroids.
6/23	Attending Physician: Platelet count continues to decrease. Will consult surgery for possible splenectomy.
	Surgical Consult: Patient examined. The risks and benefits of surgery explained and discussed. Patient is agreeable to surgery tomorrow morning.
6/24	Surgeon's Note:
	Preop Dx: ITP
	Postop Dx: Same plus cirrhosis of the liver due to alcohol use
	Procedure: Splenectomy
	Anes: GET
	Patient developed respiratory distress following extubation in the recovery room. Currently in ICU. Ventilator managed by anesthesia.
	Anesthesia: The patient currently in ICU developed very rapid shallow breathing postop and became combative. The patient was given Valium and he began to calm. The patient has decreased urinary output. Will increase IV to 125 cc/hr.
	Anesthesia: The patient is currently breathing on his own via endotracheal tube. Will return in p.m. to extubate the patient.
	Attending Note: The patient is now extubated and resting comfortably. Continue to monitor.
6/25	House Physician: Called to the floor to examine this 74-year-old male, postop one day. He was found unresponsive on the floor. There were no pulses or respirations. Code called, however, was unsuccessful. The patient was pronounced at 4:45 a.m.
	Attending Physician: The patient's course discussed with the patient's family. Condolences expressed.

PHYSICIAN'S ORDERS—PATIENT 11

DATE	ORDER
6/22	Attending MD:
	Patient admitted for treatment of ITP
	2 units of platelets
	Gamma globulin
	Type and cross 2 units PRBCs
	Tenormin 25 mg q.d.
	Prednisone 40 mg b.i.d.
	Humulin 70/30 24 units b.i.d.
	VS q. 3 hours
	BS q. 2 hours
6/23	Attending MD:
	Consult Surgery re: Splenectomy
	Surgery:
	NPO after 6 p.m.
	FBS done before OR
	Valium 20 mg in a.m.
	Decrease insulin to 12 units for evening and preop dose
6/24	Surgery:
	Admit to ICU
	Postop respiratory distress
	Vent settings as per anesthesia
	½ NSS 80 cc/hr
	Transfuse 2 units PRBCs
	Daily FBS
	Anesthesia:
	Transfer patient to floor
6/25	Release body to coroner

OPERATIVE REPORT—PATIENT 11

DATE: 6/24

PREOPERATIVE DIAGNOSIS: Idiopathic thrombocytopenic purpura

POSTOPERATIVE DIAGNOSIS: Same

OPERATION: Splenectomy

ANESTHESIA: General endotracheal

OPERATIVE INDICATIONS: Uncontrolled decreasing platelets

OPERATIVE PROCEDURE: The patient was brought to the operating room where he was placed in the supine position and prepped and draped in the usual manner. Following the induction of anesthesia, an incision was made. The abdominal cavity was entered. The liver was also found to be cirrhotic. A splenectomy was performed and the patient closed.

The patient tolerated the procedure well and was sent to the recovery room in stable condition.

PATHOLOGY REPORT—PATIENT 11

DATE: 6/24

SPECIMEN: Spleen

CLINICAL DATA: 74-year-old male with ITP

DIAGNOSIS: Spleen with increased megacaryocytes indicative of ITP

LABORATORY REPORTS—PATIENT 11

HEMATOLOGY

DATE: 6/22

Specimen	Results	Normal Values
WBC	5.0	4.3-11.0
RBC	4.3 L	4.5-5.9
HGB	12.5 L	13.5-17.5
HCT	39 L	41-52
MCV	91	80-100
MCHC	47	31-57
PLT	19 L	150-450

HEMATOLOGY

DATE: 6/23

Specimen	Results	Normal Values
WBC	5.0	4.3-11.0
RBC	4.3 L	4.5-5.9
HGB	12.5 L	13.5-17.5
HCT	39 L	41-52
MCV	91	80-100
MCHC	47	31-57
PLT	17 L	150-450

HEMATOLOGY

DATE: 6/24

Specimen	Results	Normal Values
WBC	5.0	4.3-11.0
RBC	4.0 L	4.5-5.9
HGB	11.6 L	13.5-17.5
HCT	35 L	41-52
MCV	91	80-100
MCHC	47	31-57
PLT	19 L	150-450

CHEMISTRY—PATIENT 11

Specimen	Results			Normal Values
	6/22	6/23	6/24	
GLUC	115 H	118 H	125 H	70–110
BUN	20	18	27 H	8–25
CREAT	1.0	1.0	1.0	0.5–1.5
NA	138	140	130L	136–146
K	4.0	4.5	5.4	3.5–5.5
CL	100			95–110
CO_2	30			24–32
CA	9.0			8.4–10.5
PHOS	3.0			2.5–4.4
MG				1.6–3.0
T BILI				0.2–1.2
D BILI				0.0–0.5
PROTEIN				6.0–8.0
ALBUMIN				5.0–5.5
AST	65 H	64 H	65H	0–40
ALT	79 H	82 H	77H	30–65
GCT				15–85
LD				100–190
ALK PHOS				50–136
URIC ACID				2.2–7.7
CHOL				0–200
TRIG				10–160

RADIOLOGY REPORT—PATIENT 11

DATE: 6/22

DIAGNOSIS: ITP

EXAMINATION: Chest x-ray

Heart size and shape are acceptable. The lung fields are clear and the pulmonary vascular pattern is unremarkable. There is no free fluid and the trachea remains midline.

IMPRESSION: Unremarkable chest x-ray

Enter ten diagnosis codes and three procedure codes.

PDX	
DX2	
DX3	
DX4	
DX5	
DX6	
DX7	
DX8	
DX9	
DX10	
PP1	
PR2	
PR3	

INPATIENT RECORD
DISCHARGE SUMMARY—PATIENT 12

DATE OF ADMISSION: 1/27 **DATE OF DISCHARGE:** 1/29

DISCHARGE DIAGNOSIS: Nonrheumatic congestive heart failure

ADMISSION HISTORY: This is a 57-year-old married white gentleman, referred because of recurrent shortness of breath and cough. He states that he was in his usual state of good health until approximately Christmas, when he developed a persistent cough with associated dyspnea. His dyspnea was most prominent with exertion. He was treated with Ceclor at that time, with some improvement. However, his symptoms recurred and he underwent a second course of antibiotics, again with some improvement. However, his symptoms have now recurred and he is referred for further evaluation.

He has known tricuspid insufficiency, mild left ventricular dysfunction and left ventricular dilatation by echocardiogram done 6/2. He had a normal stress ECG 10/3. The patient also has hypertension.

COURSE IN HOSPITAL: The patient was referred because of recurrent shortness of breath and cough. Apparently the patient had been doing well up until Christmas. His cough was treated with antibiotics with some improvement. His symptoms, however, recurred, requiring a second course of antibiotics.

The patient was admitted with a diagnosis of congestive heart failure. He was started on diuretics with improvement in his physical examination and his symptoms. An echocardiogram was performed, which is described as above.

The patient was extremely anxious to go home and thought that the rest of his care could be accomplished as an outpatient. He is tolerating his medications and will remain on the Capoten and the Lasix and will have a follow-up appointment with his doctor in one to two weeks and I will see him again in approximately 4 weeks. It is recommended at that time that discussion for cardiac catheterization be carried out. This was discussed with the patient during his hospitalization, the reason being that perhaps his aortic insufficiency is more significant than what is appreciated on physical examination and by echocardiogram. The catheterization would aid in the evaluation of the etiology of his LV dysfunction and his left ventricular enlargement. He has also been given information about smoking cessation.

INSTRUCTIONS ON DISCHARGE:

1. Capoten 12.5 mg b.i.d.
2. Lasix 40 mg daily
3. Insulin Humulin N 14 in a.m. with 6 of regular and Humulin N 20 units in the p.m. with 12 of regular

HISTORY AND PHYSICAL EXAMINATION—PATIENT 12

ADMITTED: 1/27

REASON FOR ADMISSION: This is a 57-year-old married white gentleman, referred because of recurrent shortness of breath and cough. He states that he was in his usual state of good health until approximately Christmas, when he developed a persistent cough with associated dyspnea. His dyspnea was most prominent with exertion. He was treated with Ceclor at that time with some improvement. However, his symptoms recurred and he underwent a second course of antibiotics, again with some improvement. However, his symptoms have now recurred and he is referred for further evaluation.

He has known moderate tricuspid valve insufficiency, mild left ventricular dysfunction and left ventricular dilatation by echocardiogram. He had a normal stress ECG on 10/3.

PAST MEDICAL HISTORY: The patient has a history of type 1 diabetes mellitus. He believes that his most recent cholesterol reading was lower than 200. He previously has been hospitalized for pericarditis and for resection of popliteal artery aneurysm. He has a history of hypertension.

ALLERGIES: None known

CHRONIC MEDICATIONS: Humulin Insulin 6 units of R and 14 units of N in the morning and 12 units of R and 20 units of N in the evening. Lotensin 20 mg PO daily.

He denies any drug allergies.

FAMILY HISTORY: Noncontributory

SOCIAL HISTORY: The patient is married and lives with his wife and smokes one to two packs of cigarettes per day.

REVIEW OF SYSTEMS: Otherwise noncontributory

HISTORY AND PHYSICAL EXAMINATION—PATIENT 12

PHYSICAL EXAMINATION: Reveals a blood pressure of 140/80, pulse 80 and regular. The patient was a pleasant, adult, white male who is in no acute distress. His carotids were without bruits. The jugular venous pulse was normal. Examination of his lungs was remarkable for fine, bibasilar rales. On auscultation of his heart, he has a regular rhythm, a soft murmur consistent with tricuspid insufficiency. Abdominal examination was unremarkable except for the presence of a liver edge just below the costal margin. He had no peripheral edema.

LABORATORY DATA: Thyroid function tests were within normal limits. Total cholesterol level was 194. His HDL and LDL are presently still pending. His blood sugar levels have been well controlled in the low 100s. His electrolytes and SMA 12 are normal as well as his complete blood count.

His EKG on admission revealed sinus rhythm with left atrial enlargement, nonspecific ST-T wave abnormality with poor R wave progression, no acute changes.

His echocardiogram revealed left ventricular enlargement, normal left atrial size at 4 cm, mild overall reduction of left ventricular contractility with diffuse hypokinesis, mild to moderate tricuspid insufficiency.

IMPRESSION:

1. Persistent shortness of breath and cough—possible nonrheumatic congestive heart failure; rule out persistent respiratory tract infection
2. Tricuspid insufficiency, left ventricular dysfunction/dilatation, by echocardiogram
3. Type 1 diabetes mellitus
4. Smoking history

CONSULTATION—PATIENT 12

DATE: 1/28

Podiatric consultation was requested. The patient's chart was reviewed in the following manner: H & P, Labs, progress notes, physician's orders, previous consultations and any other pertinent information remaining in the patient's chart.

CHIEF COMPLAINT: Diabetic foot care

PHYSICAL EXAMINATION: The patient is a 57-year-old white male admitted with a history of hypertension and diabetes mellitus, insulin dependent for approximately 7 years. The patient has shortness of breath and is a smoker. The patient states that he has had a problem with one of the valves in his heart for approximately 3 years. The patient had resection of an aneurysm in the right leg in 1989. The patient has no known drug allergies. Multiple nails, right and left feet are hypertrophic and mycotic with ingrowing tendencies. The patient has had trauma to both the great toenails at the age of 12 years due to a vehicular accident. Gait analysis will be deferred at this time. Pulses are present in both feet and ankles. The toes are warm. There are no digital lesions at this time. The muscle tone and power are fair. The patient denied having intermittent claudication during gait or phlebitis affecting either lower extremity. The patient does have some numbness of the right great toe, status post surgery for the popliteal aneurysm.

IMPRESSION:

1. Type 1 diabetes mellitus
2. Congestive heart failure
3. Valvular heart disease
4. Smoker
5. Status post resection of aneurysm of the right leg
6. Hypertension

PLAN: Podiatric consultation; initial; comprehensive. Debridement of hypertrophic mycotic nail plates bilateral feet—symptomatic

PROCEDURE: Debridement of hypertrophic mycotic nail plates, bilateral feet, symptomatic

RECOMMENDATIONS: Diabetic foot care q. 1 to 3 months. The patient will be followed p.r.n.

PROGRESS NOTES—PATIENT 12

DATE	NOTE
1/27	Physical examination reveals rales and evidence of valvular heart disease. Will diurese with Lasix and obtain an echocardiogram.
1/28	Patient better today—no shortness of breath, no edema. The importance of smoking cessation was discussed with the patient.
1/29	Will discharge the patient today.

PHYSICIAN'S ORDERS—PATIENT 12

DATE	ORDER
1/27	Chest x-ray Monitor input and output Lasix 40 mg IV now and 40 mg PO in a.m. Schedule patient for an echocardiogram CBC Consult podiatry for diabetic foot care Lotensin 20 mg PO daily in a.m.
1/23	Discharge patient to home.

LABORATORY REPORTS—PATIENT 12

HEMATOLOGY

DATE: 1/27

Specimen	Results	Normal Values
WBC	10	4.3-11.0
RBC	5.0	4.5-5.9
HGB	16.2	13.5-17.5
HCT	48	41-52
MCV	93	80-100
MCHC	35	31-57
PLT	339	150-450

RADIOLOGY REPORT—PATIENT 12

DATE: 1/28

Chest x-ray

DIAGNOSIS: The examination is compared to a prior examination on March 2 of last year. The cardiac silhouette remains at the upper limits of normal in size. The pulmonary vascularity appears slightly congested and there is a right-sided pleural effusion that was not present on the prior examination. There is minimal blunting of the left costophrenic angle. The appearance suggests congestive heart failure.

IMPRESSION: Findings of congestive heart failure

Enter seven diagnosis codes and two procedure codes.

PDX	
DX2	
DX3	
DX4	
DX5	
DX6	
DX7	
PP1	
PR2	

INPATIENT RECORD
DISCHARGE SUMMARY—PATIENT 13

DATE OF ADMISSION: 10/21 **DATE OF DISCHARGE:** 10/22

DISCHARGE DIAGNOSIS: Retained products of conception with vaginal bleeding following dilation and curettage (D & C) for miscarriage and tobacco and alcohol abuse.

COURSE IN HOSPITAL: The patient was admitted to the emergency department due to fainting and vaginal bleeding. The patient was taken to the OR for D & C. Pathology revealed desidua and chronic villa. She previously underwent a D & C for a miscarriage last week at another institution. The patient was encouraged to decrease her alcohol intake and to stop smoking. The patient appeared depressed over her recent miscarriage. A psych consult was ordered.

INSTRUCTIONS ON DISCHARGE: If heavy bleeding occurs, contact my office immediately. A follow-up visit is scheduled with the psychiatrist in 2 weeks. The patient was also given information about Alcoholics Anonymous as well as a prescription for Wellbutrin to be taken as directed for depression and smoking cessation.

HISTORY AND PHYSICAL EXAMINATION—PATIENT 13

ADMITTED: 10/21

REASON FOR ADMISSION: Heavy bleeding from vagina

HISTORY OF PRESENT ILLNESS: She has had irregular spotting and light flow on and off since a spontaneous abortion that occurred last week. She was admitted to another hospital at that time and underwent a D & C. The patient noted heavy bleeding today. She fainted in the bathroom and was brought to the emergency department by her family.

PAST MEDICAL HISTORY: The patient developed bronchitis as a child, but was not treated other than with decongestant. Her last menstrual period was 6 weeks ago.

ALLERGIES: None known

CHRONIC MEDICATIONS: None

FAMILY HISTORY: Mother has hypertension. Two sisters have had heart surgery for congenital heart problems.

SOCIAL HISTORY: The patient smokes one pack of cigarettes per day and reports intake of one 6-pack every few days during the week. The patient tried to abstain from alcohol during her pregnancy but was not successful.

REVIEW OF SYSTEMS: The patient is normally healthy. She has had a runny nose for about two days. Her bowel movements are normal, once every 2 to 3 days and her urinary function is normal. She eats three meals per day. She gets heartburn when she eats spicy foods. She drinks with her meals and into the evening on a continual basis.

PHYSICAL EXAMINATION:

HEENT: PERRL, EOM normal, thyroid not enlarged

CHEST: Clear to P & A without CVA tenderness

HEART: NSR without murmur

ABDOMEN: Soft and nontender with active bowel sounds

EXTREMITIES: Without edema, cyanosis, or clubbing

NEURO: CN's II–XII grossly intact. Reflexes are normal. No sensory or motor defects noted.

PELVIC: Uterus is of normal size with AV and femoral adnexa negative. Vaginal vault filled with serum fluid and clots. Cervix reveals pink with blood oozing from OS—no foreign body or laceration noted.

ASSESSMENT: Dysfunctional uterine bleeding

PLAN: D & C

CONSULTATION—PATIENT 13

PSYCH CONSULT

Thank you for requesting a consult with this patient. I met with her and found her to be depressed secondary to recent miscarriage. There was no evidence of suicidal thoughts. She denies any thoughts of harming herself or others. The patient has a history of alcohol abuse, three 6-packs of beer per week, and tobacco 1 ppd.

IMPRESSION:

1. Depression—secondary to recent miscarriage
2. Alcohol abuse
3. Tobacco abuse

Will treat with Wellbutrin 150 mg PO daily × 3 days then BID thereafter. Follow up in 2 weeks.

PROGRESS NOTES—PATIENT 13

DATE	NOTE
10/21	The patient has been bleeding for approximately 1 week utilizing at least 3 pads per day for flow of blood. We will repeat the D & C to determine if the patient has retained products of conception. **PREOPERATIVE DIAGNOSIS:** Severe menorrhagia **POSTOPERATIVE DIAGNOSIS:** Same **OPERATION:** Dilatation and curettage **ANESTHESIA:** Paracervical block using 1% Xylocaine and sedation using IV Valium The patient tolerated the procedure well. Await pathology report. The patient appears depressed, will order a psych consult.
10/22	The patient has decreased bleeding with decreased cramping. Will discharge today. Psych consult appreciated. The importance of decreasing alcohol and tobacco use was stressed as was the effect of these substances on fetal development. The patient will follow up with the psychiatrist after discharge.

PHYSICIAN'S ORDERS—PATIENT 13

DATE	ORDER
10/21	Admit the patient to the labor and delivery floor Vaginal prep 1,000 cc LR NPO Type and screen CBC Psych consult
10/22	Discharge patient to home

OPERATIVE REPORT—PATIENT 13

DATE: 10/21

PREOPERATIVE DIAGNOSIS: Severe menorrhagia

POSTOPERATIVE DIAGNOSIS: Same

OPERATION: Dilatation and curettage

ANESTHESIA: Paracervical block using 1% Xylocaine and sedation using IV Valium

OPERATIVE PROCEDURE: The patient was brought to the operating room and placed in the supine position. After IV Valium sedation, the patient was placed in the lithotomy position. The vaginal and perineal areas were then prepped and draped in the usual manner for vaginal surgery. Weighted speculum was inserted and the anterior retractor was used to expose the cervix. The cervix was then grasped using the Jacob's tenaculum. The paracervical block was then performed and then using Pratt dilators, the cervix was dilated up to #23. The uterus was then sounded and found to be approximately 7.5 cm. Using a medium sized sharp curette, the uterine cavity was then curetted in systematic fashion from 12 o'clock clockwise to 6 o'clock and then from 12 o'clock counterclockwise to 6 o'clock. Endometrial tissue obtained was sent to pathology. The Jacob's tenaculum was removed and with assurance of hemostasis, the weighted speculum was removed. The patient tolerated the procedure and anesthesia well and arrived in the recovery room in satisfactory condition.

PATHOLOGY REPORT—PATIENT 13

DATE: 10/22

GROSS DESCRIPTION: Labeled "endometrium" are multiple irregular fragments of tan-white tissue and blood clots, forming a spheroid 1.0 cm in diameter. All blocked.

MICROSCOPIC DESCRIPTION:

DIAGNOSIS: Secretory endometrium, with necrotic fragments of decidua and chorionic villi, consistent with retained products of conception.

LABORATORY REPORTS—PATIENT 13

HEMATOLOGY

DATE: 10/21

Specimen	Results	Normal Values
WBC	10	4.3-11.0
RBC	5.0	4.5-5.9
HGB	13.5	13.5-17.5
HCT	41	41-52
MCV	93	80-100
MCHC	35	31-57
PLT	339	150-450

Enter five diagnosis codes and one procedure code.

PDX

DX2

DX3

DX4

DX5

PP1

CCS
Answer Key

Introduction

Case-mix Exercise

1. The pyelonephritis (590.80) has a weight of 0.7864 whereas dehydration (276.51) has a weight of 0.6916. In this case, the pyelonephritis used as principal results in a higher-paying MS-DRG. This is appropriate based on the coding guideline II.C: *Two or more diagnoses that equally meet the definition for principal diagnosis* (Brown 2011, 29).
2. Using the pneumonia code first in sequence (486) has a weight of 0.7096 whereas congestive heart failure (428.0) has a weight of 1.4943. The MS-DRG 0291, HEART FAILURE & SHOCK W MCC has a higher weight (Medicare Grouper Version 28-10/10).
3. Escherichia coli pneumonia (482.82) has a weight of 1.4887 whereas COPD with acute exacerbation (491.21) has a weight of 01.1924. The bacterial pneumonia MS-DRG has a higher weight (Medicare Grouper Version 28-10/10).
4. CM = 0.7864 + 0.7096 + 1.4887 = 2.9847, CMI = 2.9847 / 3 = 0.9949. The case mix can be determined by multiplying the relative weight of each MS-DRG by the number of discharges within that MS-DRG. The sum of all the weights is the case mix. Dividing the case mix by the total number of MS-DRGs is the case-mix index (LaTour and Eichenwald Maki 2010, 436).

E/M Mapping Exercise

1. Diagnosis: 786.59, 305.1 (HHS 2010, Section IV, H).
2. CPT code using map 1—no meds given (5 points), history is PF (10 points), examination is EPF (15), tests are 5 (15 points), and supplies are none (points equal 0). Total points = 45. There were both radiology and lab tests done. CPT is 99283–25. The mapping method would be used and every hospital can develop a unique method (Clark 2009, 72–73).

Coding Exercises

Inpatient

1. 550.90, 042, 53.02 (Schraffenberger 2011, 81, 197, 202).
2. 276.51, 438.82, 787.20 (Schraffenberger 2011, 112, 169).
3. 303.00, 571.2, 305.40, 94.68 (Schraffenberger 2011, 129, 132).
4. 345.90, 350.1 (Schraffenberger 2011, 139).
5. 486,427.31—In accordance with the UHDDS, both conditions are not equally treated. The pneumonia was treated with IV antibiotics. This diagnosis had greater utilization of resources of medications and staff time compared with the atrial fibrillation, which was treated with oral medication. Because of this, the pneumonia is sequenced first (HHS 2010, Section II, C).
6. 574.10, 575.8, V64.41, 51.22 (Schraffenberger 2011, 199; HHS 2010, Section I, 18. a, 14).

7. 592.0, 591, 56.0 (Schraffenberger 2011, 210).
8. 707.07, 715.36, 707.20, 86.22 (Schraffenberger 2011, 245).
9. 722.10, 80.51 (Schraffenberger 2011, 254).

10a. 656.61, 666.02, V27.0, 72.1 (Schraffenberger 2011, 226–235).

10b. V30.00 (Schraffenberger 2011, 262, 362–363).

11. V32.01, 765.14, 773.1, 765.26 (Schraffenberger 2011, 262, 362–363).
12. 414.01, 411.1, 37.22, 88.57. The clinical scenario is one typical of unstable angina (*Coding Clinic* 5th issue, 1993, 17–24). Coronary artery disease is coded as principal (*Coding Clinic* 2nd Quarter 2004, 3; Schraffenberger 2011, 159–161).
13. 162.5, 198.3, 32.49 (Schraffenberger 2011, 94–95).
14. 198.5, 199.1 (Schraffenberger 2011, 99–101).
15. 197.7, V10.3, V45.71 (Schraffenberger 2011, 99–101).
16. 823.31, 822.0, 79.26 (Schraffenberger 2011, 291–294).
17. 969.4, 963.0, 780.2, E853.2, E858.1. The patient took over-the-counter medications with a prescription medication without consulting the prescribing physician. This is a poisoning. Per the *Official ICD-9-CM Guidelines for Coding and Reporting,* I, C, 17, e, 2, c: Nonprescribed drug taken with correctly prescribed and properly administered drug: If a nonprescribed drug or medicinal agent was taken in combination with a correctly prescribed and properly administered drug, any drug toxicity or other reaction resulting from the interaction of the two drugs would be classified as a poisoning (*Coding Clinic* 2nd Quarter 2002; HHS 2010, Section I, 17, e; Schraffenberger 2011, chapters 20 and 21).
18. 996.64, 038.11, 995.91 (Schraffenberger 2011, 320).
19. ICD: 769; CPT: 31601 (Smith 2011, chapter 4; *Coding Clinic* 1986 Nov.–Dec., 6; 1989 1st Quarter, 10).

Ambulatory/Outpatient

20. ICD: 786.59; CPT: 91034 (Schraffenberger 2011, 280; CPT Assistant May 2005, 3).
21. ICD: V76.12; CPT: 77057 (*Coding Clinic* 2003 2nd Quarter, 3–5; 2005 2nd Quarter, 2010; *CPT Assistant* March 2007, 7).
22. ICD: 173.1; CPT: 11642–E1 (Schraffenberger 2011, 95–96).
23. ICD: 735.0; CPT: 28293–TA (Schraffenberger 2011, 255; *CPT Assistant* Dec. 1996, 6; *CPT Assistant* Jan. 2007, 31).
24. ICD: 197.2 183.0; CPT: 32650 (Schraffenberger 2011, chapter 5; *CPT Assistant* Fall 1994, 1, 6; *CPT Changes: An Insider's View 2002*).
25. ICD: 427.81, 427.89; CPT: 33213; 33233 (Schraffenberger 2011, 165; *CPT Changes: An Insider's View 2003; CPT Assistant* Summer 1994, 10, 19; *CPT Assistant* Nov. 1999, 16; *CPT Changes: An Insider's View 2000*).
26. ICD: 456.1; CPT: 43243 (Schraffenberger 2011, chapter 10; *CPT Assistant* Spring 1994, 4).

27. ICD: 600.00; CPT: 52601 (Schraffenberger 2011, 212; *CPT Assistant* Nov. 1997, 20; CPT Assistant April 2001, 4; *CPT Assistant* June 2003, 6).
28. ICD: 222.1; CPT: 54056 (Schraffenberger 2011, chapter 5; Smith 2011, 121).
29. ICD: 626.8; CPT: 58563 (Schraffenberger 2011, chapter 13; *CPT Assistant* Nov. 1999, 28; March 2000, 10; March 2002, 11; *CPT Changes: An Insider's View 2000, 2002*).
30. ICD: 654.53; CPT: 59871 (Schraffenberger 2011, chapter 14; *CPT Assistant* Nov. 1997, 22; *CPT Assistant* Nov. 2006, 21; *CPT Assistant* Feb. 2007, 10).

Practice Questions

Domain 1

1. c The patient is discharged with hemiplegia and aphasia. These conditions in addition to the acute cerebral infarction should be coded (Brown 2011, chapter 24).
2. b When a patient has pulmonary edema that is due to congestive heart failure, only the congestive heart failure should be coded (Brown 2011, chapter 24).
3. b The CPK elevation with MB enzymes elevated and the EKG ST changes denote a possible MI (Brown 2011, chapter 24).
4. d Symptoms are not coded when a definitive diagnosis is present on discharge. The patient has a discharge diagnosis of urinary tract infection. The organism (*E. coli*) is coded with a secondary diagnosis code (041.4) which is to be added as an additional code to identify the bacterial agent (*Coding Clinic* 1st Quarter 1998, 5; *Coding Clinic,* July–August 1984, 19).
5. a When the attribution of a complication is uncertain, it is appropriate to query the physician (Brown 2011, chapter 4).
6. b The symptoms provided are indicative of a depressive disorder (Brown 2011, 137).
7. c The patient has abdominal adhesions with obstruction, lysis of adhesions, and the abdominal pain is not coded as it is a symptom. (*Coding Clinic* Nov.–Dec. 1987; *Coding Clinic* Jan.–Feb. 1987; *Coding Clinic* 1990 4th Quarter, 18–19; *Coding Clinic* 1995 3rd Quarter, 6; *Coding Clinic* 1995 4th Quarter, 55; Schraffenberger 2011, 205). Code 997.4, postoperative digestive system complications, excludes peritoneal (abdominal) adhesions codes 568.0 and code 568.81. In the alphabetic index, if you look under adhesions, postoperative, you will also find that 568.0 is used. Because of this, we assign 568.81 for abdominal adhesions with obstruction.
8. c Patient is found to have dysphagia with aspiration (DRG 179: Pneumonitis due to inhalation of food and vomitus) Using 486, Medicare DRG Assigned: 195 SIMPLE PNEUMONIA & PLEURISY W/O CC/MCC MDC: 04 DRG Weight = 0.7096 vs. Using 507.0, Medicare DRG Assigned: 179 RESPIRATORY INFECTIONS & INFLAMMATIONS W/O CC/MCC MDC: 04 DRG Weight = 0.9861 (Medicare Grouper Version 28-10/10).
9. d There may be endometrial implants throughout the pelvic cavity which may attach to various anatomic structures such as the fallopian tube, ovary, and omentum. These locations should be identified so that the appropriate diagnostic codes can be assigned and the appropriate procedure codes can be assigned based on the destruction of the endometrial implants. So the correct answer is to review the operative report to determine what procedure codes to use and to determine the site or sites of endometriosis so that codes with the highest specificity may be assigned and use the diagnosis of infertility as a secondary condition (*Coding Clinic* 1st Quarter 1995; *CPT Assistant* 1999; *Coding Clinic* March 2000; Schraffenberger 2011, chapter 13; Brown 2011, 227).

Domain 2

10. a Poisoning codes for aspirin and heparin and subcutaneous hemorrhage of the thigh of the right lower extremity as secondary conditions. The poisoning codes are sequenced ahead of the manifestation codes (Brown 2011, 436; HHS 2010, Section I, 17, e, 2; *Coding Clinic* 4th Quarter 1995.) Review Coding Guideline I, C, 17, e, 2, c for additional information.

11. c Code 996.01 pertains to mechanical complications and would not be used. In this case, we have pain due to the electrode. Category 996.7 is the location for pain due to devices. Please look under the heading of 996.7 in the tabular index and you will find the list of what is covered in this category. The breast cyst (610.0) would not be coded because it does not meet the criteria of the UHDDS as a secondary condition; it is an incidental finding (Brown 2011, 97–99). Code V45.79 is not added as an additional diagnosis. Review the Alphabetic Index under "Absence, thyroid, with hypothyroidism," which directs the coder to code 244.0.

12. b The abdominal pain and diarrhea are not coded as they are symptoms integral to the diagnosis of infectious gastroenteritis (Brown 2011, chapter 9).

13. c The circumstances of the encounter are for a screening colonoscopy, because of this the screening colonoscopy is listed first, followed by a code for the polyps (*Coding Clinic* 2nd Quarter 2005, 16–17).

14. a The Includes notes direct what types of neoplasms should be assigned to category 216 (Brown 2011, 17). Includes notes in category 216 specify the use of these codes (HHS 2010).

15. b The Excludes notes direct what types of neoplasms should not be assigned to category 216 (Brown 2011, 17–18). Excludes notes in category 216 specify the use of these codes (HHS 2010).

16. b The patient has mature senile cataracts, diabetes mellitus (with no designated causal relationship to the cataracts), hypertension, acute renal failure. The hypertension is not related to the renal failure as it is acute and not chronic. Because of this, a combination code for hypertension and chronic renal failure is not coded (*Coding Clinic* 3rd Quarter 1991; *Coding Clinic* 2nd Quarter 1992; Brown 2011, 123–126, 172, 221).

17. d Acute exacerbation is coded as 491.21. The hypertension is present with the chronic renal disease. Because of this, a combination code for hypertension and chronic renal disease is coded. In addition, the type of kidney disease and stage are coded (Brown 2011, 186–188, 220–222; *Coding Clinic* 4th Quarter 2006).

18. a The patient was admitted and treated for the respiratory failure. The other conditions present are also coded (Brown 2011, 189–191; *Coding Clinic* 1st Quarter 2005).

19. d The patient has cirrhosis of the liver with resulting bleeding esophageal varices. Under subcategory 456.2, see the note *Code first underlying cause, as:* Cirrhosis of liver (571.0–571.9). Because of this note, the cirrhosis is sequenced first followed by the code for the bleeding esophageal varices, followed by the code for the bleeding esophageal varices (Brown 2011, 203; *Coding Clinic* May–June 1984).

20. b The physician may word the delivery as "normal" but the coder cannot use 650 unless the patient meets the criteria for using it. The patient has a nuchal cord around the

baby's neck which precludes the use of 650 (HHS 2010, Section I, C, 11; Brown 2011, chapter 20).

21. c Codes must reflect the twin gestation as well as early delivery (Brown 2011, chapter 20).

Domain 3

22. d In order to determine the correct procedure code the lengths of the wounds repaired with the same closure are added together (AMA 2011, Surgery/Integumentary Section directions).

23. d The patient has a fracture of the right proximal ulna and the reduction does not require open reduction. In the *ICD-9-CM* book, under Fracture, ulna, proximal, the coder is referred to Fracture, ulna, upper end. The term "manipulation" is used to indicate reduction in CPT (AMA 2011, 114).

24. b A code for the anterior ethmoidectomy is assigned and to denote the bilateral procedure, a modifier of –50 is required (*CPT Assistant* Winter 1993, 23; Jan. 1997, 4; Sept. 1997, 10; Oct. 1997, 5; Dec. 2001, 6; May 2003, 5).

25. c In contrast to question 24, the code description for the transbronchial biopsy includes the specification that the biopsy is in a single lobe. An additional CPT code is needed (as opposed to a modifier) to denote the bilateral aspect of the biopsy. CPT code 31632 is an "add-on" code, which means that it is coded in addition to the primary procedure code (AMA 2011, 157–158; *CPT Assistant* 2005; May 2008, 15; Feb. 2010, 6; April 2010, 5).

26. b 37.23, 88.53, 88.56. Both the diagnostic cardiac catheterization and the cardiac angiography procedures are assigned (Brown 2011, 355; *Coding Clinic* 2005 2nd Quarter, 10–11).

27. a The procedure code assigned is associated with the diagnosis of missed abortion (Brown 2011, 300; *Coding Clinic* 3rd Quarter 1993, 6).

28. b Modifier –50 would not be used as this modifier pertains to paired organs only (*CPT Assistant* Feb. 2000, 4; Nov. 2008, 11; Oct. 2009, 12).

29. c Both the extraction of the cataract and the insertion of the lens are included in the single CPT code. The –RT modifier should be used to indicate that the right eye was involved (*CPT Assistant* Nov. 2003, 10; March 2005, 11; Sept. 2009, 5).

30. a Three codes are needed to capture the initial hour and the two additional hours. Modifier –51 would not be used in this case as modifiers are not used with add-on codes (96415) (*CPT Assistant* Nov. 2005, 1; Jan. 2007, 3; May 2007, 3; Sept. 2007, 3; Dec. 2007, 15; Feb. 2009, 17).

31. b The code for a complete chest x-ray includes a minimum of four views and does not include computer-aided detection or fluoroscopy (*CPT Assistant* July 2007, 6; Dec. 2009, 14).

32. c The localization and aspiration require two codes to identify both radiological guidance and the procedure itself (*CPT Assistant* March 2007, 7).

33. b The code that best fits the ligation is the fulguration because there are no clips or excision or lesion completed during the procedure (*CPT Assistant* Nov. 1999, 29; March 2000, 10).

Domain 4

34. c The fifth digit of "1" is used to indicate the initial episode of care for the myocardial infarction. It is used for both Hospital A as well as Hospital B as the care for the acute infarction continued with the transfer to Hospital B for a definitive procedure (Brown 2011, chapter 24; *Coding Clinic* 4th Quarter 2007, 162–167; *Coding Clinic* 3rd Quarter 2007, 10).

35. c In the inpatient setting, Rule Out diagnoses are coded as if they exist. In this case the patient has chest pain and the reason for the chest pain is rule our esophagogastroesophageal reflux disease (GERD). This requires that the GERD be coded as the first listed diagnosis (Brown 2011, 57).

36. d The ventilator management is the procedure that will impact the MS-DRG to provide appropriate reimbursement. The MS-DRG with the highest weight is 870 (Medicare Grouper Version 28-10/10).

    Ventilator management for 106 consecutive hours (96.72). Medicare DRG assigned: 870 SEPTICEMIA OR SEVERE SEPSIS W MV 96+ HOURS MDC: 18 DRG Weight = 05.8305.

    Incorrect answer option explanations provided for clarity:

    a Bronchoscopy with biopsy (33.24) reference: Medicare DRG Assigned: 872 SEPTICEMIA OR SEVERE SEPSIS W/O MV 96+ HOURS W/O MCC MDC: 18 DRG Weight = 01.1545 (*incorrect*)

    b Debridement of nails (86.27) reference: Medicare DRG Assigned: 872 SEPTICEMIA OR SEVERE SEPSIS W/O MV 96+ HOURS W/O MCC MDC: 18 DRG Weight = 01.1545 (*incorrect*)

    c Nonexcisional debridement of skin ulcer with abrasion (86.28) reference: Medicare DRG Assigned: 872 SEPTICEMIA OR SEVERE SEPSIS W/O MV 96+ HOURS W/O MCC MDC: 18 DRG Weight = 01.1545 (*incorrect*)

37. c Metastatic carcinoma of the brain; history of carcinoma of the prostate. The patient does not have a current cancer of the prostate however is being admitted and treated for metastatic cancer (to the brain, from the prostate) (HHS 2010, section I, C, 2, b).

38. a The conditions residual effects that the patient has been discharged with are coded in addition to the cerebral infarction. For code 342.91, the fifth digit of "1" is used to identify that the infarction and hemiplegia is on the left side of the brain which affects the right side of the body in this right-handed patient (Brown 2011, chapter 24).

39. c The diagnosis after study (lung cancer) was present on admission as well as the symptom (hemoptysis) (Brown 2011, Appendix A; HHS 2010, Appendix 1).

Domain 5

40. c The surgery is done on two distinct body systems with two distinct approaches. This warrants the use of –59 (*CPT Assistant* Sept. 2001).

41. d A modifier would not be assigned because the bronchus is not a paired organ. Paired organs include ears, eyes, nostrils, kidneys, lungs, ovaries, and such. (*CPT Assistant* May 2003).

42. c The melanoma is code to the site of the lesion and the procedure code is determined based on the size of the lesion as well as the margins (Brown 2011, chapter 25; *CPT Assistant* Fall 1995, 3; May 1996, 11; Nov. 2002, 5; Feb. 2010, 3).

43. b The bleeding is included in the code for diverticulosis and therefore a second code is not warranted (*CPT Assistant* 4th Quarter 1990, 20–24).

44. b The patient has a recurrent hernia with obstruction and this is captured in the diagnosis code (Brown 2011, chapter 16; *CPT Assistant* Nov. 1999, 24; March 2000, 9).

45. d The fracture code also includes the time of unconsciousness. The E codes are provided here as part of the review; however, no E codes are use on the exam except those for poisonings and adverse effects of drugs (Brown 2011, chapters 8 and 26). (Also see the Coding Instructions (for the Exam) in the Introduction of this book.)

Domain 6

46. c A combination code is not used as the renal failure is acute rather than chronic. Acute kidney failure is not the same as chronic kidney disease (Brown 2011, 220).

47. d Per *CPT Assistant,* "Codes 52234–52240 should only be reported once, regardless of the number of tumors removed. Only one of the three codes may be reported per session. Select the code based on the largest tumor. Note that 52234 is used when one or more of the tumors is under 2.0 cm and 0.5 cm or larger. Code 52240 is used when one or more of the tumors are larger than 5.0 cm" (AMA August 2009, 6).

48. d Both are types of prospective payment systems (CMS 2008).

49. c $10 \times 2.0 + 10 \times 1.5 + 10 \times 1.0 / 30 = 1.5$ The case mix can be determined by multiplying the relative weight of each MS-DRG by the number of discharges within that MS-DRG. The sum of all the weights is the case mix. Dividing the case mix by the total number of MS-DRGs is the case-mix index (LaTour and Eichenwald Maki 2010, 436).

50. a The MS-DRG weight is higher than the other MS-DRG weights and therefore the associated MS-DRG pays the most (Johns 2011, 323).

Domain 7

51. a The cancer registry can be used to undertake studies in addition to reporting cases to a central registry (LaTour and Eichenwald Maki 2010, 333).

52. c The diagnostic index can be used with the cancer registry data to undertake data quality analysis (LaTour and Eichenwald Maki 2010, 331–333).

53. a Several data sources can assist the process of improving data quality in this scenario (LaTour and Eichenwald Maki 2010, chapter 12).

Domain 8

54. a Only records that are required for care or are authorized by the patient can be released by the urgent care facility to the acute-care facility (LaTour and Eichenwald Maki 2010, chapter 10).

55. d Only conditions or procedures that are supported by documentation can be coded (LaTour and Eichenwald Maki 2010, chapter 11).

56. d Disclosing information without the patient's written consent violates the patient's right to privacy (LaTour and Eichenwald Maki 2010, chapter 10).

57. d Health information should not be left in public view (LaTour and Eichenwald Maki 2010, chapter 10).

Domain 9

58. d Only those conditions that are documented by the physician should be coded (LaTour and Eichenwald Maki 2010, chapter 11).

59. d If a procedure is performed, the operative report provides a detailed discussion of what was done (LaTour and Eichenwald Maki 2010, chapter 10).

60. b In order to code the procedure accurately, specific information must be documented and used to assign the code (Brown 2011, chapter 24).

PRACTICE—PATIENT 1

PDX	550.90	Left inguinal hernia
DX2	214.4	Lipoma of spermatic cord (as per path. and operative reports)
PP1	49505-LT	Hernia repair
PR2	55520-59	Excision lipoma

Notes for Practice Outpatient Case—Patient 1

550.90 The type of hernia is coded (Brown 2011, 208–209).

214.4 The lipoma is also removed and so should be coded (Brown 2011, 377–378).

49505–LT The hernia location is on the left and the laterality is reported (*CPT Assistant* Sept. 2000, 10).

55520–59 The lipoma requires excision and is therefore coded (*CPT Assistant* Sept. 2000, 10).

PRACTICE—PATIENT 2

PDX	338.4	Chronic pain syndrome
DX2	724.4	Lumbar radiculopathy
PP1	62311	Injection, single (not via indwelling catheter), not including neurolytic substances, with or without contrast (for either localization or epidurography), of diagnostic or therapeutic substance(s) (including anesthetic, antispasmodic, opioid, steroid, other solution), epidural or subarachnoid; lumbar, sacral (caudal)

Notes for Practice Outpatient Case—Patient 2

338.4 The patient has a diagnosis of chronic pain syndrome and a code from the 338.category should be assigned. Per the *Official ICD-9-CM Guidelines for Coding and Reporting* I, C, 6, 1, a: "Category 338 codes as principal or first-listed diagnosis." Category 338 codes are acceptable as principal diagnosis or the first-listed code when pain control or pain management is the reason for the admission/encounter. The underlying cause of the pain should be reported as an additional diagnosis, if known (Brown 2010, 163; *Coding Clinic* 2nd Quarter 2007, 14).

724.4 This code denotes the specific cause of the pain (Brown 2011, chapter 9).

62311 *CPT Assistant* states "62311 should only be coded once" (AMA Nov. 2008).

PRACTICE—PATIENT 3

PDX	338.3	Pain management
DX2	174.8	Breast cancer of left upper breast
DX3	198.5	Metastatic bone CA
PP1	62362	Implantation programmable pump for pain management

Notes for Practice Outpatient Case—Patient 3

338.3 The patient is admitted for pain management due to metastatic cancer .If the admission is for pain control related to , associated with, or due to, a malignancy, code 338.3 (Brown 2011, 163; *Coding Clinic* 2nd Quarter 2007, 13–14).

174.8, 198.5 The primary site and metastatic sites should be coded (Brown 2011, 378–382).

62362 The reservoir is surgically placed and attached to a previously placed catheter (*CPT Assistant* March 1997, 11).

PRACTICE—PATIENT 4

PDX	337.22	Reflex sympathetic dystrophy, left knee
PP1	64520-LT	Left lumbar sympathetic block with C-arm
PR2	77003	Fluroscopic guidance and localization of needle or catheter tip

Notes for Practice Outpatient Case—Patient 4

337.22 The diagnostic code is needed to establish the medical necessity for the procedure and a pain management code is not appropriate because the underlying condition is being treated (Brown 2011, 163).

64520–LT When coding paravertebral spinal nerves and branches, it is appropriate to use the modifiers to note the laterality (*CPT Assistant* July 1998, 10; April 2005, 13).

77003 Fluroscopic guidance is not included in the 64520 code so it is therefore appropriate to code a second code (*CPT Assistant* March 2007, 7; July 2008, 9; Feb. 2010, 12).

PRACTICE—PATIENT 5

PDX	182.0	Endometrial carcinoma
DX2	998.2	Accidental laceration
DX3	998.0	Postoperative shock
DX4	285.1	Acute blood loss anemia
DX5	280.0	Chronic blood loss anemia
DX6	244.0	Post-surgical hypothyroidism
DX7	998.11	Intraoperative hemorrhage
DX8	568.81	Hemoperitoneum
DX9	V16.0	Family history of colon cancer
PP1	68.51	Laparoscopic assisted vaginal hysterectomy
PR2	39.31	Suture of lacerated epigastric artery

Notes for Practice Inpatient Case—Patient 5

182.0	Endometrial carcinoma is documented in the pathology report and the discharge summary (Brown 2011, 379–382).
998.2	Accidental laceration is documented in the second operative report (Brown 2011, 453). In the 998 category, a coder may double code—one code to denote the complication and the other to provide specificity. In other instances, only one code is needed. 998.2 is a general complication code. Adding an additional code notes what organ was lacerated.
998.0	Postoperative shock is denoted in the discharge summary (Brown 2011, 453). Include this because there is no other code to denote postoperative shock. Only one code is used.
285.1	Acute blood loss anemia is documented in the progress notes and operative report because the patient had blood loss of 1,500 to 2,000 mL. The labs also reflect this diagnosis (*Coding Clinic* 2nd Quarter 1992).
280.0	The patient also had chronic blood loss anemia as documented on the H & P (*Coding Clinic* 4th Quarter 1993).
244.0	Postsurgical hypothyroidism is documented on the H & P report and patient received Synthroid while an inpatient (Brown 2011, 132).
998.11	Intraoperative hemorrhage documented in the operative report (Brown 2011, 453). 998.11 is a general complication code; the coder does not know where the hemorrhage is taking place. By adding an additional code, a coder can indicate where the hemorrhage is occurring.
568.81	Coded to add further specificity (Brown 2011, 453).
68.51	The patient underwent a laparoscopic-assisted vaginal hysterectomy. (Do not code the laparoscopy because it is the operative approach.) (Brown 2011, 68).
39.31	The patient underwent another laparoscopy for suture of the lacerated epigastric artery. (Do not code the laparoscopy because it is the operative approach.) (Brown 2011, 68).

Note: Chronic cervicitis is not coded because it is an incidental finding (Brown 2011, 99).

Note: Based on the following instructions for the CCS exam (refer to the Introduction of this book), the blood transfusion is not coded: Do not code procedures that fall within the code range 87.01–99.99. But, code procedures in the following ranges:

87.51–87.54	Cholangiograms
87.74, 87.76	Retrogrades, urinary systems
88.40–88.58	Arteriography and angiography
92.21–92.29	Radiation therapy
94.24–94.27	Psychiatric therapy
94.61–94.69	Alcohol/drug detoxification and rehabilitation
96.04	Insertion of endotracheal tube
96.56	Other lavage of bronchus and trachea
96.70–96.72	Mechanical ventilation
98.51–98.59	ESWL
99.25	Chemotherapy

Practice Exam 1

1. c The American Thoracic Society has defined status asthmaticus as an acute asthmatic attack in which the degree of bronchial obstruction is not relieved by the usual treatment, such as by epinephrine or aminophylline (*Coding Clinic* 4th, Quarter 1988, 9–10).

2. c Unfortunately, urosepsis is sometimes stated as the diagnosis even though the condition has progressed to a septicemia in which a localized urinary tract infection has entered the blood stream and become a generalized sepsis. The physician should be asked if the diagnosis of urosepsis is intended to mean (1) generalized sepsis (septicemia) caused by leakage of urine or toxic urine by products into the general vascular circulation, or (2) urine contaminated by bacteria, bacterial by products, or other toxic material but without other findings (Brown 2011, 110).

3. b It is rare for only one coronary artery to be bypassed, and it is also fairly common to perform both an internal mammary-coronary artery bypass and an aortocoronary bypass at the same operative episode (Schraffenberger 2011, 174).

4. c A colonoscopy is an examination of the entire colon, from the rectum to the cecum that may include the terminal ileum. In general, a colonoscopy examines the colon to a level of 60 cm or higher (Smith 2010, 117).

5. c Herceptin therapy is not antineoplastic chemotherapy, but is a biological adjuvant treatment for women with breast cancers that are HER2 positive. Herceptin is a type of targeted cancer therapy also referred to as a monoclonal antibody (*Coding Clinic* 3rd Quarter 2009, 26(3):3).

6. a When the attending physician does not confirm the results of the radiology report for inpatient coding, query the attending physician regarding the clinical significance of the findings and request that appropriate documentation be provided (*Coding Clinic* 2nd Quarter 2002, 17). This is an example of a circumstance where the chronic condition must be verified. All secondary conditions must meet the UHDDS definitions; it is not clear if COPD does (*Coding Clinic* 1st Quarter 2004, 21(1):20–21).

7. d Coding strictly from the pathology report is not appropriate as the coder is assigning a diagnosis without the attending physician's corroboration. It is therefore appropriate to query the physician. (*Coding Clinic* 1st Quarter 2004, 2(1):20–21).

8. c Excisional debridement can be performed in the operating room, the emergency department, or at the bedside. Coders are encouraged to work with the physician and other healthcare providers to ensure that the documentation in the health record is very specific regarding the type of debridement performed. If there is any question as to whether the debridement is excisional or nonexcisional, the provider should be queried for clarification (Schraffenberger 2011, 249).

9. b When a patient is readmitted because a complication has developed following discharge for a treated miscarriage, a code from category 639 is assigned as the principal diagnosis. The 639 code is used because the miscarriage (spontaneous abortion) was dealt with in a prior episode of care (Schraffenberger 2011, 223).

10. d Code 414.01 is assigned to show coronary artery disease in a native coronary arteryandis used when a patient has coronary artery disease and no history of coronary bypass graft (CABG) surgery (Schraffenberger 2011, 159–162; AMA *CPT Professional Edition* 2011, 481–482). 93458 is a new code for 2011 and includes intraprocedural injection(s) for left ventricular/left atrial angiography, imaging supervision, and interpretation when performed (AMA *CPT Professional Edition* 2011, Cardiac Catheterization Guidelines, 482).

11. a Common reasons for revision joint replacement surgery include mechanical loosening of the prosthesis, dislocation of the prosthetic joint, fracture of the bone around the implant. To classify mechanical reasons for revision joint replacement, ICD-9-CM diagnosis codes 996.40–996.49 are provided. In addition to one of these codes, the patient should also be assigned a code from the V43.60–V43.69 range to identify the joint previously replaced by prosthesis. The note in the tabular procedure index directs the coder to add an additional code for the type of bearing surface. Revision of the acetabular component involves removal and exchange of the entire acetabular component, including both the metal shell and the polyethylene, ceramic, or metal modular bearing surface. Common indications for acetabular component revision are wear of the modular bearing surface, aseptic loosening, malposition of the component, or infection (Schraffenberger 2011, 319; *Coding Clinic* 3rd Quarter 1997, 14(3):13).

12. b When an admission involves delivery, the principal diagnosis should identify the main circumstance or complication of the delivery. The 650 code cannot be used because there is a complication of pregnancy because the pregnancy is prolonged. The difference between 645.11 and 645.21 is that 645.1x represents more than 40 completed weeks to 42 completed weeks while 645.2x represents gestation of beyond 42 weeks (Schraffenberger 2011, 226, 229; *Coding Clinic* 4th Quarter 2000, 17(4):43).

13. b ICD-10-CM was developed under the leadership of the National Center for Health Statistics (NCHS), a federal agency under the Centers for Disease Control (CDC). Full compliance is expected for claims received for encounters and discharges occurring on or after 10/1/2013 (Brown 2011, 464).

14. a Pseudoaneurysm usually occurs at the site of previous vascular surgery or vessel puncture, which occurs secondary to a rent or defect in the vessel. The vessel was intentionally punctured in order to accomplish the procedure. This type of problem should not be assigned to code 998.2, Accidental puncture or laceration during a procedure (*Coding Clinic* 3rd Quarter 2002, 19(3):24–27).

15. d Patients with acute ischemic heart disease or acute myocardial ischemia does not always indicate an infarction. It is often possible to prevent infarction by means of surgery and/or the use of thrombolytic agents if the patient is treated promptly. If there is occlusion or thrombosis of the artery without infarction, code 411.81, Acute coronary occlusion without myocardial infarction, is assigned (Brown 2011, 337; *Coding Clinic* 3rd Quarter 1989, 6(3):4–5).

16. d Nausea, vomiting, and abdominal pain are symptoms of acute cholecystitis. Signs and symptoms that are associated routinely with a disease process should not be assigned as additional codes, unless otherwise instructed by the classification (HHS 2010, Section I, B, 7).

17. c If the findings are outside the normal range and the attending provider has ordered other tests to evaluate the condition or prescribed treatment, it is appropriate to ask the provider whether the abnormal findings should be added Abnormal findings from laboratory, x-ray, pathologic, and other diagnostic results are not usually coded and reported unless the physician indicates their clinical significance (Brown 2011, 99).

18. b Code 458.2, Iatrogenic hypotension, should be assigned to describe this condition. This code should be assigned when hypotension develops as a result of any type of medical care. Assign code E941.2, Sympathomimetics (adrenergics), to indicate that it is an adverse effect of the drug (*Coding Clinic* 3rd Quarter 2002, 19(3):12).

19. b A tear in the dura that occurs during spinal surgery is not unusual and is typically repaired intra-operatively when identified. Primary closure of the dural tear is usually accomplished. Dural tears that are not discovered during surgery can result in leakage of cerebrospinal fluid (CSF), leading to CSF headache, caudal displacement of the brain, subdural hematoma, spinal meningitis, pseudomeningocele and/or a dural cutaneous fistula (*Coding Clinic* 4th Quarter 2008, 109–110).

20. a Respiratory failure may be listed as a secondary diagnosis if it occurs after admission, or if it is present on admission, but does not meet the definition of principal diagnosis (Brown 2011, 189–191; *Coding Clinic* 2nd Quarter 2000, 17(2):22).

21. b Code 481, Pneumococcal pneumonia, is assigned when both conditions exist. Code also 038.2, Pneumococcal septicemia as well as the SIRS (*Coding Clinic* 1st Quarter 1999, 13; HHS 2010, Section I, C, 1, b, 2, a).

22. b Patients who have undergone kidney transplant may still have some form of CKD, because the kidney transplant may not fully restore kidney function. Therefore, the presence of CKD alone does not constitute a transplant complication. Assign the appropriate 585 code for the patient's end stage renal disease and code V42.0 (HHS 2010, Section I, C, 10, a, 2).

23. c Incorporating internal and external auditing into the coding compliance plan has proven to be the best strategy. Internal auditing enables managers to see first-hand where their units' strengths and weaknesses lie. External auditing provides an unbiased view of a department's performance. Together, internal and external audits help coding managers build effective education plans for their units (Castro and Layman 2011, 43).

24. d Before any unlisted code is assigned, the coding professional should review HCPCS Level II (national) codes to confirm that CMS has not developed a specific code for the procedure or service in question. CPT Category III codes, which are developed specifically for reporting new technology, should also be reviewed. CPT guidelines support the use of a Category III code instead of a Category I unlisted code (Smith 2011, 23).

25. a CT colonography uses CT scanning to obtain an interior view of the colon (the large intestine) that is otherwise only seen with a more invasive procedure where an endoscope is inserted into the rectum (Kuehn 2011, 157). *Note:* Code 0066T has been deleted and the coder is instructed to use 74263. Computed tomographic (CT) colonography, screening, including image postprocessing (AMA *CPT Professional Edition* 2011, 370).

26. c 11602: Excision malignant lesion of trunk . . . excised diameter 1.1 cm to 2.0 cm. The size of the lesion plus the margins are included in coding the excision. Excised diameter: 1.0 cm + 0.2 cm + 0.2 cm = 1.4 cm (Smith 2010, 55–57).

27. c Assign code 80.59, Other destruction of intervertebral disc, for the procedure performed. IDET involves only the disc not the nerve root. IDET is done with thermal energy (heat) directed into the outer disc wall (annulus) and inner disc contents (nucleus) via a heating coil, decreasing the pressure inside the disc. Code 04.2, Destruction of cranial and peripheral nerves, would not be the correct code assignment, because it relates to the peripheral nerves (*Coding Clinic* 3rd Quarter 2002, 10).

28. c For tubal ligation, which may be performed by ligation, transaction, or other occlusion of the fallopian tubes, the coder should refer to codes 58600–58615 for abdominal or vaginal approaches. For laparoscopic tubal ligation with the use of Falope rings, code 58671 is assigned (Kuehn 2011, 182).

29. c Codes (52234–52240) should only be reported once, regardless of the number of tumors removed. Only one of the three codes may be reported per session. Select the code based on the largest tumor. Code 52240 is used when one or more of the tumors are larger than 5.0 cm (*CPT Assistant* August 2009, 19(8):6).

30. c A variety of substances can be injected into the submucosal space of the digestive tract through a sheathed needle-tipped catheter inserted through an endoscope (*CPT Assistant* May 2005, 15(5):3–6).

31. c The endometrial biopsy (58110) is an add-on code and there are specific directions in the CPT book to use this code in conjunction with the code for the colposcopy; *(CPT Changes 2006—An Insider's View; CPT Assistant* June 2006, 16–17).

32. c CPT code 52204 is reported only once, irrespective of how many biopsy specimens are obtained and how the specimens are sent for pathologic examination (*CPT Assistant* August 2009, 19(8):6).

33. d The operative report should be reviewed for the body part involved with the lesion. The total size of the excised area, including margins, is needed for accurate coding. The pathology report typically provides the specimen size rather than the lesion or excised size. Because the specimen tends to shrink, this is not an accurate measurement according to the intent of the code assignment (Smith 2011, 56–57).

34. c The blood gas values of pO_2 of 58, pCO_2 of 55, pH of 7.32 reflect respiratory failure and the patient was treated in ICU with intubation and mechanical ventilation DRG: 0207, RESPIRATORY SYSTEM DIAGNOSIS W VENTILATOR SUPPORT 96+ HOURS. The addition of procedure codes for the intubation and ventilation would move this to MS-DRG 207. The acute exacerbation of COPD with blood gas values of pO_2 of 58, pCO_2 of 55, pH of 7.32 reflects possible respiratory failure. The patient was treated with intubation and mechanical ventilation for more than 96 hours. MS-DRG 0207 is a correct reflection of the patient's severity illness and appropriate reimbursement resulting based on the documentation when compared to the MS-DRG associated with acute exacerbation of COPD (491.21), which is MS-DRG 192 (weight: 0.7222) (Medicare Grouper Version: 28-10/10).

35. b MS-DRG 291 (weight: 1.4943) for congestive heart failure with stage III pressure ulcer would optimize the MS-DRG. MS-DRG 293 (weight: 0.6853) is assigned for congestive heart failure alone, with atrial fibrillation, with blood loss anemia, and with coronary artery disease all remain the same (Medicare Grouper Version 28-10/10).

36. d MS-DRG 264 (weight 2.5305) for myocardial infarction with transbronchial lung biopsy would result in the highest reimbursement. MS-DRG 316 (weight: 06147) would be assigned for the myocardial infarction alone, and with insertion central venous catheter. MS-DRG 282 (weight: 0.8064) would be assigned for myocardial infarction with mechanical ventilator (Medicare Grouper Version 28-10/10).

37. d The principal diagnosis should be the condition established after study that was responsible for the patient's admission. If the patient was admitted with a condition that resulted in the performance of a cesarean procedure, which condition should be selected as the principal diagnosis? If the reason for the admission/encounter was unrelated to the condition resulting in the cesarean delivery, the condition related to the reason for the admission/encounter should be selected as the principal diagnosis, even if a cesarean was performed (HHS 2010, Section I, C, 11, b, 4).

38. d This patient was previously treated for the spontaneous abortion but the presence of the products of conception denotes that the abortion was not completed during the prior episode of care. Because of this and the fact that she now has sepsis, she is coded as having an incomplete spontaneous abortion with sepsis (Brown 2011, 294).

39. a MS-DRG 314 (weight: 1.8145) for myocardial infarction with respiratory failure would optimize the MS-DRG. MS-DRG 316 (weight: 0.6147) would be assigned for myocardial infarction alone, with atrial fibrillation, with hypertension, and with history of myocardial infarction (Medicare Grouper Version 28-10/10).

40. c Payment status indicators that are assigned to an APC and indicate APC payment are G, H, K, P, R, S, T, U, X, and V. Status indicator N denotes that there is no specific payment for that APC because the procedure payment is included in another APC. There may be multiple APCs with the same or different payment status indicator per claim. In this case, all APCs impact payment except the one with status indicator N (Casto and Layman 2011, 185).

41. d Multiple surgical procedures with payment status indicator T performed during the same operative session are discounted. The highest-weighted status T procedure is fully reimbursed. All other procedures with payment status indicator T are reimbursed at 50%. In this case there is only one status T procedure and it is paid 100% (Casto and Layman 2011, 183).

42. a Multiple surgical procedures with payment status indicator T performed during the same operative session are discounted. The highest-weighted procedure is fully reimbursed. All other procedures with payment status indicator T are reimbursed at 50%. Because of this, if another T procedure were codes, it would be reimbursed at 50% (Casto and Layman 2011, 183).

43. d The codes are differentiated according to the route of administration. For Medicare cases, a Level II HCPCS code (J series) is reported with the identification of the specific substance or drug; for non-Medicare cases, code 99070 may be reported. In this case, use both 96372 and J0570. *Note:* HCPCS codes are used in the multiple choice questions but are not assigned when coding the cases on the CCS exam (Smith 2011, 237–238). Refer to the Coding Instructions (for the Exam) in the Introduction of this book.

44. d Several tools and references are used to support the reimbursement process including the fee schedule and the current National Correct Coding Initiatives edits. Other valuable resources are Medicare's Carrier Manual, Medicare's National Coverage Determinations Manual, and local coverage determinations (LCDs) (Hazelwood and Venable 2011, 292).

45. a The UHDDS item 11-b defines *other diagnoses* as "all conditions that coexist at the time of admission, that develop subsequently or that affect the treatment receive d and/or the length of stay (HHS 2010, Section III).

46. b The OCE has four basic functions: editing the data on the claims for accuracy, specifying the action the FI should taken when specific edits occur, assigning APCs to the claim (for hospital outpatient services), and determining payment-related conditions that require direct reference to HCPCS codes or modifiers. Routine edits for age and sex are done on all claims (Smith 2011, 261).

47. c The *case mix* is defined as a methods of grouping patients. MS-DRGs are often used to determine case mix in hospitals. The *case-mix index* is the average MS-DRG weight based on the specific patient group and is determined by multiplying the DRG weights by the number of patients and then divided by the total number of patients: 30 + 20 + 10 = 60 / 30 = 2.0 (LaTour and Eichenwald Maki 2011, 436).

48. a MS-DRG 195 (weight: 3.0) Simple pneumonia and pleurisy age >17 w/CC results in higher reimbursement than MS-DRG 193 (weight: 2.0) Simple pneumonia without MCC or CC (Medicare Grouper Version 28-10/10).

49. d In the paper chart, a line can be drawn through an erroneous entry, initialed, and the correction made along the margin. In an electronic record, the correction may be placed in the wrong sequence, which may adversely impact patient care (Johns 2011, 183).

50. c For reporting purposes the definition for *other diagnoses* is interpreted as additional conditions that affect patient care in terms of requiring: clinical evaluation; or therapeutic treatment; or diagnostic procedures; or extended length of hospital stay; or increased nursing care and/or monitoring (HHS 2010, Section III).

51. c Data mining is associated with data warehouses. *Data mining* is a process that identifies patterns and relationships by searching through large amounts of data. Because data warehouses contain large amounts of data, data mining processes are frequently used to systematically analyze these data. In healthcare, data mining is used to identify methods for cutting healthcare costs, suggest more appropriate medical treatments, and predict medical outcomes (Johns 2011, 910).

52. c *DRG groupers* are software programs that help coders determine the appropriate diagnosis-related group (DRG) assignment based on the logic of the system for hospital inpatients. APC groupers are software programs that help coders determine the appropriate ambulatory payment classification for an outpatient encounter (Johns 2011, 449).

53. a An *information system* (IS) consists of data, people, and work processes and a combination of hardware (machines and media), software (computer programs), and communication technology (computer networks) known as information technology (IT) (Johns 2011, 876).

54. c Reviewing the history and physical of a coworker when not part of assigned work is not ethical because the review is not part of designated work. This violates the ethical principal of acting with integrity and behaving in a trustworthy manner (AHIMA 2004; Schraffenberger 2011, 509).

55. a The HIM professional must know the retention statutes and retention periods in his or her state of employment (LaTour and Eichenwald Maki 2011, 282).

56. b The role of the *risk manager* is to collect and analyze information on actual losses and potential risks and to design systems that lessen potential losses in the future. An incident report is a structured tool used to collect data and information about any event not consistent with routine operational procedures (Johns 2011, 653).

57. a *Coding compliance policies* serve as a guide to performing coding and billing functions and provide documentation of the organizations' intent to correctly report services. The policies should include facility-specific documentation requirements, payer regulations and policies, and contractual arrangements for coding consultants and outsourcing services. This information may be covered in payer/provider contracts or found in Medicare and Medicaid manuals and bulletins (AHIMA 2008, 83–88).

58. b As of August 17, 2000, HHS published the final regulations for electronic transactions and coding standards as established under HIPAA in the *Federal Register* (65 FR 50312; Schraffenberger 2011, xiv).

59. d When a symptom is followed by contrasting/comparative diagnoses, the symptom is sequenced first. All the contrasting/comparative diagnosis should be coded as additional diagnoses (HHS 2010, Section II, E).

60. b *External cause of injury codes* are used to provide information about how an injury occurred, the intent (intentional or unintentional), provide information about where the injury occurred, and the status of the person at the time the injury occurred. In the case of a person who seeks care for an injury or other health condition that resulted from an activity, or when an activity contributed to the injury or health condition, activity codes are used to describe the activity (Brown 2011, 400–402).

EXAM 1—PATIENT 1

PDX	233.0	Carcinoma in situ of breast
PP1	19301-RT	Mastectomy, partial (eg, lumpectomy, tylectomy, quadrantectomy, segmentectomy)
PR2	38525	Biopsy or excision of lymph node(s); open, deep axillary node(s)
PR3	38792	Injection procedure; for identificaion of sentinel node

Notes on Patient 1

233.0 This is an example of carcinoma in-situ of the breast. By looking up the morphologic type of carcinoma, in situ, intraductal of specified site in the Alphabetic Index, the coder is directed to "see neoplasm, by site, in situ (Brown 2011, 377).

19301–RT The patient underwent a lumpectomy. The modifier –RT is also important because the breast is a paired organ (*CPT Assistant* Feb. 2007, 4; Dec. 2007, 8; Sept. 2008, 5, March 2010, 10).

38525 Sentinel lymph node dissection was undertaken (*CPT Assistant* May 1998, 10; July 1999, 7; Oct. 2005, 23; Dec. 2007, 8; Sept. 2008, 5).

38792 The injection of vital dye (eg, isosulfan blue) to visualize the sentinel node in the OR may be reported separately with code 38792 (*CPT Assistant* July 1999, 7, 12).

EXAM 1—PATIENT 2

PDX	388.10	Chronic serous otitis media, simple or unspecified
DX2	473.9	Unspecified sinusitis (chronic)
DX3	474.12	Hypertrophy of adenoids alone
PP1	69436-50	Tympanostomy (requiring insertion of ventilating tube), general anesthesia (bilateral)
PR2	42831	Adenoidectomy, primary; age 12 or over (Patient is 35 years old.)

Notes on Patient 2

381.10 The patient has chronic serous otitis media (the specific documentation of "serous otitis media" is found in the postoperative diagnosis in the operative report) (Scraffenberger 2011, 143).

473.9, 474.12 The patient also has chronic sinusitis and adenoid hypertrophy (Brown 2011, chapter 15).

69436–50 The patient had a bilateral tympanostomy. The modifier –50 is used to identify the bilateral procedure (rather than listing the procedure code twice).

42831 The patient also had adenoidectomy. This code is affected by age.

EXAM 1—PATIENT 3

PDX	371.23	Bullous keratopathy
DX2	379.31	Aphakia
DX3	365.10	Open-angle glaucoma, unspecified
DX4	364.10	Chronic iridocyclitis, unspecified
DX5	413.9	Other and unspecified angina pectoris
DX6	496	Chronic airway obstruction (COPD)
PX1	65750-LT	Keratoplasty (corneal transplant); penetrating (in aphakia)
PR2	66985-LT	Insertion of intraocular lens prosthesis (secondary implant), not associated with concurrent cataract removal
PR3	67010-LT	Removal of vitreous, anterior approach (open sky technique or limbal incision); subtotal removal with mechanical vitrectomy

Notes on Patient 3

371.23, 379.31, 365.10, 364.10	The conditions specified in the record should be coded (Brown 2011, 169–173).
413.9	Angina should be coded as it meets the UHDDS definition of another diagnosis (Brown 2011, 338).
496	COPD should be coded as it meets the UHDDS definition of another diagnosis (Brown 2011, 186–188).

Note: History of prostate cancer is not coded because it does not have an effect on the current encounter (Brown 2011, 90).

Note: The –LT modifier denoting the left eye is used on all of the procedure codes:

65750–LT *CPT Assistant* Oct. 2002, 8; April 2009, 5; Dec. 2009, 13

66985–LT *CPT Assistant* Sept. 2005, 12; Sept. 2009, 5

67010–LT *CPT Assistant* Fall 1992, 4

EXAM 1—PATIENT 4

PDX	872.01	Open wound of ear, auricle
PP1	12011-LT	Simple repair of superficial wounds of face, ears, eyelids, nose, lips and/or mucous membranes; 2.5 cm or less (2 cm laceration specified in the physical examination)
PR2	99283-25	E/M code based on mapping scenario provided (40 total points*)

Notes on Patient 4

872.01 The laceration is of the external ear, of the auricle.

12011-LT A simple repair of the ear was done of less than 2.5 cm (*CPT Assistant* Feb. 2000, 10; May 2000, 8; Jan. 2002, 10; Feb. 2008, 8).

99282-25 The coder will need to calculate the evaluation and management code for the outpatient visit. *According to the mapping scenario; meds given are = 1= 5 points, the history is problem focused = 10 points, the exam is problem focused = 10 points, the number of tests = 0 = 5 points, supplies = 2 suture kits = 10 points. This equals 40 points.

EXAM 1—PATIENT 5

PDX	812.21	Fracture of humerus, shaft of humerus
DX2	305.1	Tobacco use disorder
PP1	24505-LT	Closed treatment of humeral shaft fracture; with manipulation, with or without skeletal traction
PR2	99284-25	E/M code based on mapping scenario provided (50 total points*)

Notes on Patient 5

812.21 The patient has sustained a fracture of the humerus (Brown 2011, 407–409).

305.1 The patient received tobacco cessation counseling and instructions to see her primary care physician (Schraffenberger 2011, 130).

24505-LT In CPT, *reduction* is termed treatment of fracture with manipulation.

99284-25 Calculate the evaluation and management code for the outpatient visit. *According to the mapping scenario; meds given are = 2 = 5 points, the history is problem focused = 10 points, the exam is extended problem focused = 15 points, the number of tests = 5 = 15 points, supplies = 1 fracture tray = 5 points. Total is 50 points.

EXAM 1—PATIENT 6

PDX	414.01	Coronary atherosclerosis of native coronary artery
PP1	93460	Catheter placement in coronary artery(s) for coronary angiography, including intraprocedural injection(s) for coronary angiography, imaging supervision and interpretation; with right and left heart catheterization including Intraprocedural injection(s) for left ventriculography, when performed.
PR2	93567	Injection procedure during cardiac catheterization including imaging supervision, interpretation, and report; for supravalvular aortography (List separately in addition to code to code for primary procedure.)

Notes on Patient 6

414.01 The patient has arteriosclerotic heart disease with no history of cardiac bypass (Schraffenberger 2011, 160–162).

93460 Catheter placement in coronary artery(s) for coronary angiography, including intraprocedural injection(s) for coronary angiography, imaging supervision and interpretation; with right and left heart catheterization including intraprocedural injection(s) for left ventriculography, when performed (Kuehn 2011, 259).

+93567 Injection procedure during cardiac catheterization including imaging supervision, interpretation, and report; for supravalvular aortography. (List separately in addition to code to code for primary procedure.)

EXAM 1—PATIENT 7

PDX	197.7	Secondary malignant neoplasm of liver
DX2	162.5	Malignant neoplasm of lung, lower lobe
PP1	10022	Fine needle aspiration; with imaging guidance
PR2	76942	Ultrasonic guidance for needle placement (eg, biopsy, aspiration, injection, localization device), imaging supervision and interpretation

Notes on Patient 7

197.7 The patient is being seen because of the metastatic cancer of the liver (Brown 2011, 387).

162.5 The patient's primary site is the right lower lobe of the lung (Brown 2011, 387).

10022 The patient undergoes a fine needle aspiration with imaging guidance (*CPT Assistant*, Nov. 2002, 1; June 2007, 10).

76942 The ultrasound guidance is also coded (*CPT Assistant* Fall 1993, 12; Fall 1994, 2; May 1996, 3; June 1997, 5; Oct. 2001, 2; May 2004, 7; Dec. 2004, 12; April 2005, 15–16; Aug. 2008, 7; March 2009, 8).

EXAM 1—PATIENT 8

PDX	820.21	Fracture of neck of femur, intertrochanteric section
DX2	997.5	Urinary complications
DX3	788.20	Retention of urinary, unspecified
DX4	428.0	Congestive heart failure, unspecified
DX5	562.10	Diverticulosis of colon (without mention of hemorrhage)
DX6	424.0	Mitral valve disorders
DX7	414.01	Coronary atherosclerosis of native coronary artery
DX8	V12.71	History of peptic ulcer disease
DX9	715.90	Osteoarthritis, unspecified
DX10	290.0	Senile dementia, uncomplicated
PP1	79.35	Open reduction with internal fixation of femur

Notes on Patient 8

820.21 Radiology report denotes intertrochanteric fracture (Brown 2011, 407).

997.5 Patient had postoperative urinary retention as documented in the 12/1 progress note. The 997 category directs coders to use an additional code to identify the specific complication in addition to 997 (*Coding Clinic* 2nd Quarter, 1998).

788.20 Patient had postoperative urinary retention as documented in the 12/1 progress note. The 997 category directs coders to use an additional code to identify the specific complication in addition to 997(*Coding Clinic* 2nd Quarter, 1998).

428.0 Congestive heart failure (Brown 2011, 339–340).

562.10 Brown 2011, 205

424.0 Aortic valve disorder (Brown 2011, 330–332).

414.01 Arteriosclerotic heart disease (Brown, 2011, 330–332).

V12.71 Brown 2011, 83

715.90 Brown 2011, 253

290.00 Brown 2011, 135–137

79.35 Brown 2011, 410–411

Note: Per the Coding Instructions (for the Exam), "Do not code 57.94 (Foley catheter)."

Points of Interest on Patient 8

1. This case provides an example of postoperative urinary retention, which is a commonly missed complication.
2. You must review the radiology report to determine where the fracture is. This is frequently the case with coding actual records.

EXAM 1—PATIENT 9

PDX	663.31	Delivery complicated by nuchal cord without compression
DX2	V27.0	Single liveborn
DX3	648.61	Other cardiovascular diseases in the mother classifiable elsewhere, but complicating pregnancy, childbirth, or the puerperium
DX4	424.0	Mitral valve disorders
PP1	73.6	Episiotomy

Notes on Patient 9

663.31 As per the delivery note, this is a delivery with a nuchal cord wrapped around the baby's neck (Brown 2011, 289).

V27.0 Outcome of delivery code (Brown 2011, 270).

648.61, 424.0 These must be coded because they affected the monitoring of the patient and were documented in the medical record. The "use additional code" note at category 648 directs the coder to add another code to identify the condition (Brown 2011, 276–277).

73.6 Episiotomy—the repair of an episiotomy is included in the code (Brown 2011, 282).

Points of Interest on Patient 9

1. In terms of documentation, this case is typical of many delivery charts. Often times, practitioners document the complication of delivery in only one area, such as the delivery note or the operative report. In this case, the baby has a nuchal cord, but it is only mentioned once in the delivery record.
2. This is also an illustration of the three types of codes, at a minimum, that must be on every delivery chart: a diagnostic code from the delivery or pregnancy category, an outcome of birth code (V code), and a procedure code.

EXAM 1—PATIENT 10

PDX	482.83	Pneumonia due to other gram-negative bacteria
DX2	250.52	Diabetes with ophthalmic manifestations, type II or unspecified type, uncontrolled
DX3	362.01	Background diabetic retinopathy
DX4	401.9	Essential hypertension, unspecified
DX5	V09.2	Infection with microorganisms resistant to macrolides
DX6	715.36	Osteoarthritis, localized, knees
DX7	424.1	Aortic valve disorders
DX8	V58.67	Long-term (current) use of insulin

Notes on Patient 10

482.83 Gram-negative pneumonia documented on the H & P and 2/2 progress note (*Coding Clinic* 3rd Quarter, 1988).

250.52 Noninsulin-dependent diabetes mellitus (insulin requiring) used because the H & P states "Diabetes mellitus–uncontrolled" 1/31 progress note addresses treatment plan for diabetes out of control. Orders of 1/31 and 2/1 reflect treatment. The blood glucose record reflects high blood sugar (*Coding Clinic* 4th Quarter 1997; *Coding Clinic* 2nd Quarter 1997; *Coding Clinic* 2nd Quarter 2002; *Coding Clinic* 3rd Quarter 2002).

362.01 Retinopathy is documented on the discharge summary (Brown 2011, 125).

401.9 Documented on the H & P and discharge summary. The patient is on HCTZ for this condition (Brown 2011, 346–350).

V09.2 Reported because the resistant organism is documented in the discharge summary and laboratory reports. Furthermore, the patient tried erythromycin and needed to be changed to another antibiotic (Brown 2011, 113).

715.36 Documented in the D/C summary, H & P, and the orders (Brown 2011, 253–254).

424.1 Documented in the D/C summary, H & P, and the orders (Brown 2011, 330–332).

V58.67 Brown 2011, 122

Points of Interest on Patient 10

1. The patient has pneumonia and documentation needs to have the organism causing the pneumonia specified in the medical record in areas other than just the sputum culture.
2. The patient also has uncontrolled diabetes as evidenced by the labile blood sugar and the documentation in the record.
3. Coders should only use the V codes denoting resistance when the resistance is documented by the physician(s) involved (Brown 2011, 113).

EXAM 1—PATIENT 11

PDX	V58.11	Encounter for antineoplastic chemotherapy
DX2	197.6	Secondary malignant neoplasm of retroperitoneum and peritoneum
DX3	789.51	Malignant ascites
DX4	V10.05	Personal history of malignant neoplasm of large intestine
DX5	V44.3	Status colostomy
DX6	V16.0	Family history of malignant neoplasm of gastrointestinal tract
DX7	V15.3	History of radiation therapy
DX8	V15.82	History of tobacco use
DX9	V45.72	Acquired absence of intestine (large) (small)
PP1	99.25	Chemotherapy

Notes on Patient 11

V58.11 The patient is admitted for chemotherapy, as documented in the discharge summary and reflected in the physician orders (Brown 2011, 388).

197.6 Carcinomatosis with malignant ascites from retro-peritoneum and peritioneum is documented on the discharge summary and H & P (Brown 2011, 379–382).

789.51 The *ICD-9-CM* Tabular Index requires the malignancy be coded first (Brown 2011, 379–382).

V10.05 The organ of origin (colon) has been removed; therefore, code the history of malignant neoplasm of the colon. Whenever there is a secondary neoplasm code, primary site must be designated either with a code for the primary site or a V code. If the primary site for the neoplasm is not known, use code 199.1 (Brown 2011, 380).

V44.3 Status colostomy is reflected on the H & P (Brown 2011, 89).

V16.0 Relevant to the patient's treatment and documented in the medical record (Brown 2011, 83–84).

V15.3 Brown 2011, 83–84

V15.82 Brown 2011, 83–84

V45.72 The documentation indicates that a colectomy was done to treat the patient's primary colon cancer.

99.25 Per the Coding Instructions (for the Exam), this code for chemotherapy would be assigned. (For exam coding instructions, refer to the Introduction of this book.)

Note: Breast cyst is not coded because it does not meet UHDDS criteria.

Points of Interest on Patient 11

1. This case illustrates several basic principles of coding neoplasms. First, the patient had the organ in which the carcinoma arose removed (organ of origin). Second, because a secondary site is being coded, the coder must code the primary site in some manner. Therefore, use a history of malignancy code (V10.06) to represent the primary site.

2. This case also illustrates that when the ascites is determined to have malignant cells in the fluid, the code for malignant ascites should be used. Under code 789.51, there is a "code first malignancy, such as . . ." which determines the sequencing of the diagnosis codes.

EXAM 1—PATIENT 12

PDX	162.5	Malignant neoplasm of lung, lower lobe
DX2	997.1	Cardiac complications (Intraoperative myocardial infarction [MI])
DX3	410.71	Acute myocardial infarction, subendocardial infarction
DX4	401.9	Essential hypertension, unspecified
DX5	458.29	Iatrogenic hypotension
DX6	496	Chronic airway obstruction, not elsewhere classified (COPD)
DX7	721.3	Lumbosacral spondylosis without myelopathy
DX8	438.21	Hemiplegia affecting dominant side
DX9	V15.82	History of tobacco use
DX10	V15.3	History of radiation therapy
PP1	32.59	Pneumonectomy

Notes on Patient 12

162.5	Recurrent lung cancer is documented in the H & P, discharge summary, and operative report (Brown 2011, 378–382).
997.1	Brown 2011, 452
410.71	Postoperative/intraoperative myocardial infarction is documented in the progress notes (Brown 2011, 452).
401.9	Hypertension documented in the H & P and the D/C summary (Brown 2011, 346–349).
458.29	This is the precipitating factor causing the MI (Brown 2011, 352).
32.59	Pneumonectomy is documented in the operative report.
496, 721.3, 438.21	Should be coded because they are documented in the medical record and are relevant to the admission (HHS 2010, Section III, 89; Brown 2011, chapters 15, 19, 24).
V15.82	HHS 2010, Section I, c, 18, d, 4
V45.76	HHS 2010, Section I, c, 18, d, 3
32.59	Brown 2011, 89–90

Point of Interest on Patient 12

1. This case allows the coder to practice coding an intraoperative complication. Further, the coder needs to differentiate if the myocardial infarction caused the hypotension or if the hypotension caused the myocardial infarction. In this case, the intraoperative hypotension occurred, which resulted in an MI. This case illustrates that problem. This is a clinical scenario about which coders have little education.

EXAM 1—PATIENT 13

PDX	410.41	Acute myocardial infarction of other inferior wall
DX2	426.0	Atrioventricular block, complete
DX3	578.0	Hematemesis
DX4	285.1	Acute posthemorrhagic anemia
DX5	272.4	Hyperlipidemia
DX6	414.01	Coronary atherosclerosis of native artery
DX7	787.01	Nausea with vomiting
DX8	E938.4	Adverse effect of other and unspecified general anesthetics
DX9	V15.82	History of tobacco use
PP1	36.12	Aortocoronary bypass of two coronary arteries
PR2	36.06	Insertion of non-drug-eluting coronary artery stent(s)
PR3	37.22	Left heart cardiac catheterization
PR4	88.55	Coronary arteriography using a single catheter
PR5	88.53	Angiocardiography of left heart structures
PR6	45.13	Other endoscopy of small intestine (EGD)
PR7	00.66	PTCA
PR8	00.45	Insertion of one vascular stent
PR9	00.40	Procedure on single vessel
PR10	39.61	Extracorporeal circulation auxiliary to open heart surgery

Notes on Patient 13

410.41 Acute inferior MI is documented on the 4/20 EKG. This is also evident from the laboratoryreports because the CK-MB is elevated (Brown 2011, 333–334).

426.0 Complete heart block is documented on the discharge summary, the H & P, and the EKG (Brown 2011, chapter 24).

578.0 Code the hematemesis because no cause has been found (Brown 2011, 201–202).

285.1 Following the upper gastrointestinal bleeding, the patient experienced acute blood loss anemia (Brown 2011, 152).

272.4 Hyperlipidemia is documented on the H & P and summary (Brown 2011, chapter 11).

414.01 Patient is found to have arteriosclerotic heart disease. Code the native artery (fifth digit of "1") because the patient has never undergone bypass surgery prior to this admission. Therefore, assume the ASHD is of the native artery (Brown 2011, 337).

787.01 Nausea and vomiting is the adverse effect of a drug (E938.4) (Brown 2011, 435).

E938.4 Adverse effect of anesthesia (Brown 2011, 435).

V15.82 History of tobacco use (Brown 2011, 89–90).

36.12 CABG ×2 (Brown 2011, 360–364).

36.06 Insertion non-drug-eluting stents (Brown 2011, 360).

37.22 Left heart catheterizations (Brown 2011, 355).

88.55 Angiography using a single catheter (Brown 2011, 355).

88.53 Ventriculography (Brown 2011, 355).

45.13	EGD (Brown 2011, chapter 16).
00.66	PTCA
00.45	Insertion of one vascular stent
00.40	Procedure on a single vessel
39.61	Extracorporeal (Brown 2011, 360).

Points of Interest on Patient 13

1. The coder must code the site of the myocardial infarction to obtain the correct fourth digit. Look at the EKG to determine the site of acute inferior myocardial infarction. Keep in mind the coding guideline related to ST elevation myocardial infarction (STEMI) and non-ST elevation myocardial infarction (NSTEMI) (HHS 2010, Section I, 7, e, 1).
2. This case also requires a code for the upper gastrointestinal hemorrhage because there is no specified cause.
3. Recognize nausea and vomiting is an adverse effect of anesthesia.
4. The CABG and the heart catheterization provide practice in this area. Remember stents, if they are placed, by coding with an additional code when coding PTCAs. Also code the angiography and ventriculography, if done. To correctly code these procedures, carefully determine how many catheters are used during the angiography in order to code them appropriately.
5. If extracorporeal circulation is used, code this as directed by the *ICD-9-CM* codebook notation. Cardioplegia would not be coded because this is included in the coronary artery bypass code.
6. Per the Coding Instructions (for the Exam), the following procedures would *not* be coded: "Code all procedures that fall within the code range 00.01–86.99, but do not code 57.94 (Foley catheter)." Because of this direction, do not code 99.10 for the TPA. (For CCS exam coding instructions, refer to this book's Introduction.)

Practice Exam 2

Domain 1

1. a A miscarriage is a spontaneous abortion. If the readmission is for the purpose of dealing with retained products of conception, a code from the 634–637 is assigned along with the fifth digit of "1" to indicate that it was incomplete (Brown 2011, 294).

2. a Recurring mood changes that result in periods of severe depression alternating with extreme elation that are beyond the normal range of mood swings are called bipolar or circular disorders (Brown 2011, 137–138).

3. d A cesarean section is performed for a variety of reasons, such as cephalopelvic disproportion (CPD), prolapsed cord, fetal distress, and conditions of the mother. Based on the information given in this case, fetal head was measured and then it was decided a cesarean section should be performed. It is likely that the reason for this was CPD; therefore, physician should be queried (Brown 2011, 273; APA 2007; Lovaasen and Schwerdtfeger 2011, 624).

4. c With the documented clinical indicators, it would be appropriate to query the physician regarding the possibility of a complication resulting from surgery. When formulating a query, it is unacceptable to lead a provider to document a particular response. The query should not be directing or probing and the provider should not be led to make an assumption (Lovaasen and Schwerdtfeger 2011, 42).

5. d According to *Coding Clinic,* if there is evidence of a diagnosis within the medical record and the coder is uncertain whether it is a valid diagnosis because the documentation is incomplete, it is the coders responsibility to query the attending physician to determine if this diagnosis should be included (AMA 2nd Quarter 2000, 17–18).

6. b Esophageal varices are often associated with cirrhosis of the liver. In this case, dual coding is required with the underlying condition coded first. For example, esophageal varices with cirrhosis of liver is coded as 571.5 (cirrhosis of liver) + 456.21 (esophageal varices in diseases classified elsewhere) (Brown 2011, 203).

7. a An inpatient is a patient who is provided with room, board and continuous general nursing services in an area of an acute-care facility where patients generally stay at least overnight (Johns 2011, 705; Scott 2009, 3).

8. d The patient is being seen in the emergency room, which is a hospital outpatient department. Because of this, all CPT and HCPCS codes should be captured so that the correct reimbursement is obtained (Kirchoff 2009, 33–42).

9. b According to AHIMA documentation guidelines, any additional late entry to the record should be labeled as such and these addenda should be added if the physician is queried but the associated documentation to support the code assignment is not present in the original record. In this case, it is an addendum (Johns 2011, 107).

Domain 2

10. a When the diagnostic statement lists the symptom first, followed by two or more contrasting/comparative conditions, a symptom may be assigned as a principal diagnosis (Brown 2011, 29–30, 97).

11. c In this case, there is documentation of the ventilator associated pneumonia (VAP), therefore, code 997.31, Ventilator associated pneumonia, should be assigned. An additional code to identify the organism should also be assigned (041.7, Pseudomonas aeruginosa). No additional codes from categories 480–484 to identify the type of pneumonia are assigned (HHS 2010, Section I, C, 17, f, 3, a).

12. d An adverse reaction can occur when is correctly prescribed and administered. In the case of an adverse reaction, the manifestation is coded first (Hematuria) followed by an E code for the medication (Coumadin) (Schraffenberger 2010, 284; HHS 2009, Section I, C, 17, e, 1).

13. c Pleural effusion can be a symptom of CHF, however, in this case, it can be coded because it meets the definition for coding additional diagnosis (it required a diagnostic procedure and it was still unresolved at discharge (HHS 2010, Section III).

14. c This is a confirmed HIV case, therefore, it should be coded first, followed by the additional diagnosis code for all reported HIV-related conditions. Also, the scenario describes a bacterial pneumonia, therefore, code 482.41 is assigned and 484.8 is not used (HHS 2010, Section I, C, 1, a, 1–2).

15. d When assigning codes for diabetes and its associated conditions, the code(s) from category 250 must be sequenced before the codes for the associated conditions. Without additional documentation regarding the specific diabetic manifestation related to the heel ulcer, the only code choice for the diabetes is 250.80 (HHS 2010, Section I, C, 3, a, 4).

16. d Heart conditions (425.8, 429.0–429.3, 429.8, 429.9) are assigned to a code from category 402 when a causal relationship is stated (due to hypertension) or implied (hypertensive). Use an additional code from category 428 to identify the type of heart failure in those patients with heart failure (HHS 2010, Section I, C, 7, a, 2).

17. c The ICD-9-CM Neoplasm table reference at the beginning of the table provides instruction related to sites marked with the * sign. When referencing *neoplasm, knee* in the table, an * is found after *knee* NEC. The instructions direct the coder as follows: *"Sites marked with the sign * should be classified to malignant neoplasm of skin of these sites...."* Follow that path and code to neoplasm, skin, knee, and the correct answer is 173.7, Malignant neoplasm of skin, skin of lower limb, including hip (Brown 2010, chapter 25).

18. a Alphabetic Index for fracture, orbital, roof guides the coder to see fracture, skull, base. After evaluating the selections for the fourth and fifth digit, the correct answer is 801.00, Fracture of base of skull, closed without mention of intracranial injury, unspecified state of consciousness (Brown 2011, 406–407).

19. d Both burns are at the same body part, therefore, only the highest degree burn should be coded (Brown 2011, 426).

20. b An intentional drug overdose is coded as poisoning. Also, according to Schraffenberger, in poisoning cases, E codes should be assigned as necessary to completely describe the cause, intent and place of occurrence (HHS 2010, Section I, C, 17, e, 2, b; Schraffenberger 2010, 304; Brown 2011, 436).

21. d When the drug was correctly prescribed and properly administered, code the reaction plus the appropriate code from the E930–E949 series. If the specific reaction is not documented, it is appropriate to choose code 995.20 (HHS 2010, Section I, C, 17, e, 1).

Domain 3

22. a Manipulation refers to the attempted reduction or restoration of a dislocated joint or fracture (Smith 2011, 82).

23. c When multiple wounds are repaired with the same closure type (for example, simple), lengths of the wounds in the same classification and from all anatomical sites that are grouped together into the same code descriptor should be added together (Smith 2011, 65–66).

24. d A complex repair of a wound goes beyond a layer closure and requires scar revision, debridement, extensive undermining, stents, or retention sutures (Smith 2011, 65).

25. a Codes 65710–65757 are used to describe keratoplasty or corneal transplants. This case does not mention penetrating but anterior lamellar keratoplasty. Therefore, the correct code assignment is 65710, Keratoplasty (corneal transplant), anterior lamellar (*CPT Changes Insider's View* 2009).

26. c Codes 49650–49659 describe procedures related to laparoscopic hernia repairs. Note that 49657 was a new code in 2009 to specifically describe laparoscopic surgical repair of recurrent incisional hernia, incarcerated (including mesh insertion) (Smith 2011, 124).

27. b Code 50593, Ablation, renal tumor(s), unilateral, percutaneous, cryotherapy is used for cryoablation of renal tumors (AMA *CPT Professional Edition* 2011, 269).

28. c CPT codes 92980 and 92981 would be reported for transcatheter stenting of a single coronary vessel (Smith 2011, 205).

29. a Surgery is the only treatment and cure for ventral hernias and effective October 1, 2008, a new code 53.71, was added for laparoscopic repair of diaphragmatic hernia, abdominal approach (*Coding Clinic* 4th Quarter, 2008, 165–169).

30. b This episode of care occurs in the ER which is an outpatient setting, therefore, a CPT code should be used. CPT code 36831 correctly identifies the thrombectomy procedure (Kirchoff 2009, 203).

31. d A myringotomy for insertion of ventilating tubes is a tympanostomy, which is described by codes 69433–69436. Code 69436, Tympanostomy (requiring insertion of ventilating tube), general anesthesia describes the procedure performed. In addition, this procedure was performed bilaterally, therefore, modifier –50 is added (Smith 2011, 160).

32. d According to Smith, the documentation needed to properly code removal of skin tags includes diagnosis of skin tags and the number of skin tags removed. These details are provided in the scenario given, therefore, the correct code assignment is 11200, Removal of skin tags, multiple fibrocutaneous tags, any area; up to and including 15 lesions (Smith 2011, 59).

Domain 4

33. c According to the UHDDS definition of the secondary diagnosis, a secondary or additional diagnosis is the diagnosis which receives clinical evaluation, therapeutic treatment, further evaluation, extends length of stay or increases nursing monitoring/care (HHS 2010, Section II).

34. b Beginning in fiscal year 2009, CMS designated stage III and IV pressure ulcers as a hospital acquired condition (HAC). If a HAC diagnosis is present at admission (Y), it will continue to be classified as CC or MCC and will impact MS-DRG reimbursement. If a HAC diagnosis is not present at admission (N), it will no longer be classified as CC or MCC and will decrease MS-DRG reimbursement (Garrett 2009, 11).

35. c According to the UHDDS definition of the principal diagnosis is "that condition established after study to be chiefly responsible for occasioning the admission of the patient to the hospital for care." In this case, metastatic carcinoma of the brain is responsible for the patient's fall, ataxia and syncope (HHS 2010, Section II).

36. b Congestive heart failure includes symptoms such as shortness of breath and pleural effusion. Since these symptoms are the main reason for admission, congestive heart failure is the probable principal diagnosis (Schraffenberger 2011, 164).

37. a This is an instance when two diagnoses equally meet the definition of principal diagnosis, therefore, either of the diagnoses may be sequenced as principal diagnosis (HHS 2009, Section II, C).

38. a The postoperative complication that is not present at admission. The insurance company may not pay for the services provided to take care of the postoperative complication (Garrett 2009, 11).

Domain 5

39. d The outpatient code editor (OCE) performs four basic functions: editing the data on the claim for accuracy, specifying the action the fiscal intermediary should take when specific edits occur, assigning APCs to the claim (for hospital outpatient services) and determining payment-related conditions that require direct reference to HCPCS codes or modifiers. Choice "d" is not one of these functions (Smith 2011, 261).

40. d A colonoscopy is the examination of the entire colon, from the rectum to the cecum, that may include the terminal ileum (AMA *CPT Professional Edition* 2011, 243).

41. b When a patient presents for outpatient surgery, code the reason for the surgery as the first-listed diagnosis (reason for the encounter) even if the surgery is not performed due to a contraindication (HHS 2009, Section IV, A, 1).

42. d Total reimbursement is $3,300 ($2,000 for the procedure with status indicator S + $50 for the procedure with status indicator X + $1,000 for the first procedure with status indicator T + $250 for the second procedure with status indicator T). Use 50% of the reimbursement for the lower reimbursement APC with status indicator T (Casto and Layman 2011, 175–183).

43. a Multiple surgical procedures with payment status indicator T performed during the same operative session are discounted. The highest weighted procedure is fully reimbursed and all procedures with payment status indicator T are reimbursed at 50%. Procedure code 10060 is associated with the lower reimbursement APC with status indicator T, therefore, will be paid at 50% (Casto and Layman, 2011, 175–183).

44. d Status S procedures are not discounted when multiple procedures are done (Kirchoff 2009, 12).

Domain 6

45. b Outpatient prospective payment system (OPPS) is used for outpatient hospital services. A hernia repair procedure can be performed in a hospital outpatient setting, therefore, would be paid under the OPPS (Casto and Layman 2011, 4).

46. b A payment status indicator establishes how the service is paid in the hospital outpatient prospective payment methodology (Casto and Layman 2011, 175).

47. a There is only one MS-DRG per inpatient discharge but there can be one or more APCs per outpatient visit (Casto and Layman 2011, 180). (Also, refer to the exam coding instructions in the Introduction of this book for more details.)

48. c The correct answer is 45 ($2.0 \times 10 + 1.5 \times 10 + 1.0 \times 10$) Case mix is the sum of relative weights (Latour and Eichenwald Maki 2010, 436).

49. a Compare MS-DRG relative weights for DRG 191, 192, and 193. The lower the relative weight, the lower the payment. DRG 193 has the lowest weight and therefore admitting more patients in this DRG will only lower the CMI the payment is lowest for DRG 193 (Johns 2011, 323). DRG 193 has the lowest weight.

Domain 7

50. d The disease and procedure indices would be used. Such tasks are usually performed more efficiently by avoiding manual abstraction of the records and utilizing reporting capabilities built in various information systems (LaTour and Maki 2010, 331).

51. d The procedure index would be used. Such tasks are usually performed more efficiently by avoiding manual abstraction of the records and utilizing reporting capabilities built in various information systems. In addition to this, filtering the data by using the predetermined RBC values for blood transfusion, will sort out the blood transfusion cases and make the ones who did not follow the predetermined criteria easily identifiable (LaTour and Maki 2011, 331).

52. d A billing and reimbursement abstracting system tracks diagnosis and procedure codes assigned and will identify which cases to correct (LaTour and Maki 2011, 331).

Domain 8

53. c Coding tasks include review of records assigned, completion of abstracting and evaluation of coding quality but not risk analysis for medical record documentation (AHIMA 2008).

54. d Routine computer back-ups are a preventive measure and assure data saving at predetermined intervals; therefore, data loss is minimized in the event of "down time" (Johns 2011, 925–927).

55. d This question relates to the need-to-know principle. The medical staff member who is not associated with the patient's care does not need to see that patient's record (Johns 2011, 778–779).

56. a In this case, health information is being used for payment purposes, which is part of the Privacy Rule related to TPO—Treatment, Payment, and Operations (Johns 2011, 823).

Domain 9

57. c Bylaws must include a requirement that a history and physical exam must be completed and documented for each patient no more than 30 days before or 24 hours after admission or registration, but prior to surgery or a procedure requiring anesthesia services (Medicare Conditions of Participation: Medical Staff 2003, 485).

58. a Regular internal audits are an important part of the coding compliance plan. Choice "b," audits performed by external reviewers is part of the coding compliance plan but is more expensive and not done as frequently as the internal audit. Choice "c," audits performed by physician payers are not part of the coding compliance plan. Choice "d," sharing and discussing results with admission staff is part of the compliance plan but occurs after the internal audit is performed (Schraffenberger 2007, 223).

59. c Careful discharge planning ensures that proper follow up medical or nursing care after the patient leaves the hospital. This is continuity of care (Johns 2011, 652).

60 c Coding audits performed by physician payers may occur but are not part of the coding compliance plan (Davis and LaCour 2007, 156).

EXAM 2—PATIENT 1

PDX	836.1	Tear of lateral cartilage or meniscus of knee, current
DX2	844.2	Sprains and strains, cruciate ligament of knee
PP1	29881-RT	Arthroscopy, knee, surgical; with meniscectomy (medical OR lateral, including meniscal shaving)
PR2	29888-RT	Athroscopically aided anterior cruciateligament repair/augmentation or reconstruction

Notes on Patient 1

836.1 The condition requiring repair (Brown 2011, chapters 19 and 26).

844.2 An additional condition requiring surgery (Brown 2011, chapter 26).

29881–RT Code is used for the repair of the menisectomy (*CPT Assistant* Feb. 1996, 9; June 1999, 11; Aug. 2001, 7; Oct. 2003, 11; April 2005, 14; Dec. 2007, 10).

29888–RT Represents the arthroscopic repair of the ligament (*CPT Assistant* Oct. 2003, 11; Dec. 2007, 10).

EXAM 2—PATIENT 2

PDX	727.1	Bunion
PP1	28296-TA	Correction, hallux valgus (bunion), with or without sesamoidectomy; with metatarsal osteotomy (eg, Mitchell, Chevron, or concentric type procedures)

Notes on Patient 2

727.1 This is the code for a bunion and the definition for bunion can be found in *Dorland's Medical Dictionary* (Kuehn 2011, 126–128).

28296 Third-party payers require submission of CPT codes with various modifiers, such as –TA for left foot, great toe (AMA *CPT Professional Edition* 2011). This type of bunionectomy is described in the medical record (*CPT Assistant* Dec. 1996, 6; Jan. 2007, 31).

EXAM 2—PATIENT 3

PDX	493.92	Asthma with (acute) exacerbation
PP1	99284-25	E/M code based on mapping scenario provided
PR2	96365	Intravenous infusion, for therapy, prophylaxis, or diagnosis (specify substance or drug); initial, up to 1 hour

Notes on Patient 3

493.92 This condition brought the patient to the emergency department (Brown 2011, 186–187).

99284–25 This code represents the evaluation and management code for the facility APV and is done according to the mapping scenario as follows; meds given are = 2 = 5 points, the history is problem focused = 10 points, the exam is extended problem focused = 15 points, the number of tests = 4 = 15 points, supplies = one venipuncture set and one intravenous set = 10 points. 55 total points.

96365 The IV infusion is separately reportable and an additional code should be assigned (*CPT Changes: An Insider's View* 2009).

EXAM 2—PATIENT 4

PDX	789.01	Abdominal pain, right upper quadrant
DX2	787.01	Nausea with vomiting
DX3	276.51	Dehydration
DX4	530.81	Gastroesophageal reflux
DX5	300.00	Anxiety
PP1	99285-25	Evaluation and management mapping for case hospital visit level 5

Notes on Patient 4

789.01 This is the most severe symptom and the reason for the encounter (Brown 2011, 98).

787.01 This is a secondary condition that was evaluated and treated (Brown 2011, 98).

276.51 This is a secondary condition that was evaluated and treated (Brown 2011, 30).

530.81 This is a secondary condition that was evaluated and treated (Brown 2011, 203).

300.00 This is coded but does not fit within the requirements of 4 diagnoses required by the exam procedures.

99285–25 This is code is used to represent the evaluation and management code for the facility APV and is done according to the mapping scenario as follows; meds ordered are = 3 = 10 points, the history is comprehensive = 25 points, the exam is extended problem focused = 15 points, the number of tests = 6 = 20 points, supplies = 1 IV = 5 points. 75 total points.

EXAM 2—PATIENT 5

PDX	414.01	Coronary atherosclerosis of native coronary artery
PP1	92980-LD	Transcatheter placement of an intracoronary stent(s), percutaneous, with or without other therapeutic intervention, any method; single vessel
PR2	93458	Left heart catheterization including intrprocedural injections for left ventriculography, imaging supervision and interpretation

Notes on Patient 5

414.01 This is the reason for the heart catheterization (Brown 2011, chapter 24).

92980 This code identifies the insertion of the drug-eluting stent into the left anterior descending coronary artery. The stenting procedure and is not reported separately because only the most complex procedure is coded (Kuehn 2011, 257–258).

–LD The –LD modifier is used to identify that the PTCA/stent was completed in the left anterior descending coronary artery.

93458 This is a new code in 2011 for cardiac catheterization and angiography (*CPT Changes: An Insider's View* 2011, 186).

EXAM 2—PATIENT 6

PDX	338.3	Neoplasm related pain (acute) (chronic)
DX2	154.3	Malignant neoplasm, anus, unspecified
DX3	198.0	Secondary malignant neoplasm, kidney
DX4	197.0	Secondary malignant neoplasm, lung
DX5	198.3	Secondary malignant neoplasm, brain and spinal cord
DX6	401.9	Essential hypertension, unspecified
DX7	345.90	Epilepsy, unspecified (Seizure disorder NOS)
PP1	36569	Insertion of peripherally inserted central venous catheter (PICC), without subcutaneous port or pump; age 5 years or older
PR2	77001	Fluoroscopic guidance for central venous access device placement

Notes on Patient 6

338.3	The reason for the patient encounter is to manage pain due to cancer. In this case code 338.3 should be assigned. The underlying neoplasm is reported as an additional diagnosis (Brown 2011, 163).
154.3, 198.0, 197.0, 198.3	The primary site of the cancer (anal) as well as all secondary sites are coded (Brown 2011, 378–381).
401.9, 345.90	These conditions are coded because they are chronic conditions (Brown 2011, 30).
36569	This is the code for insertion of PICC line in patient age 5 and older (*CPT Assistant* Oct. 2004, 14; Dec. 2004, 8; May 2005, 13; June 2008, 8).
77001	This is coded to represent the fluoroscopic guidance (*CPT Assistant* March 2007, 7; July 2008, 9).

EXAM 2—PATIENT 7

PDX	681.10	Cellulitis and abcess, toe
DX2	707.15	Ulcer of other part of foot
DX3	355.8	Mononeuritis of lower limb, unspecified
DX4	244.9	Unspecified hypothyroidism
DX5	401.9	Essential hypertension, unspecified
PP1	10060	Incision and drainage of abscess (eg, carbuncle, suppurative hidradenitis, cutaneous or subcutaneous abscess, cyst, furuncle, or paronychia); simple or single

Notes on Patient 7

681.10 The patient has an abscess/cellulitis of the toe (Brown 2011, 242–243).

707.15 This condition is coded as it related to the abscess (Brown 2011, 242).

355.8 This condition is coded as it is a chronic condition (Brown 2011, 161).

244.9 This condition is coded as it is a chronic condition (Brown 2011, chapter 11).

401.9 This condition is coded as it is a chronic condition (Brown 2011, 346).

10060 AMA *CPT Professional Edition* 2011, 57

EXAM 2—PATIENT 8

PDX	656.41	Intrauterine death, delivered, with or without mention of antepartum condition
DX2	653.41	Fetopelvic disproportion, delivered, with or without mention of antepartum condition
DX3	663.31	Other and unspecified cord entanglement, without mention of compression, delivered, with or without mention of antepartum condition
DX4	649.11	Obesity complicating pregnancy, childbirth, or the puerperium, delivered, with or without mention of antepartum condition
DX5	278.00	Obesity, unspecified
DX6	V27.1	Single stillborn
PP1	74.0	Classical cesarean section
PR2	73.09	Other artificial rupture of membranes (not for induction of labor)
PR3	75.32	Fetal EKG (scalp)

Notes on Patient 8

663.31 Used to denote the nuchal cord without compression as documented in the operative report (Brown 2011, 281).

649.11 Obesity in pregnancy and delivery as documented in the history and physical (Brown 2011, 269).

278.00 Coded to add further specificity to category 649.11 (Brown 2011, 129).

V27.1 Outcome of delivery for stillborn code (Brown 2011, 270).

73.09 Used to denote the artificial rupture of membranes performed after Pitocin is administered and labor fails to progress as documented in the H & P (Brown 2011, 282).

75.32 Use of internal fetal monitor (Brown 2011, 282).

Note: Per the exam coding instructions (in the Introduction of this book), "Code all procedures that fall within the code range 00.01–86.99, but do not code 57.94 (Foley catheter)."

Points of Interest on Inpatient 8

1. This is an example of a very unfortunate situation of a baby's death. The intrauterine death is sequenced first because it is the reason for the cesarean section. Although it was thought the patient had cephalopelvic disproportion, the urgency of undertaking the cesarean section was due to the lack of fetal heart tones.
2. Code 73.4 is not assigned because it is not documented. In practice, the coder would query the physician.

EXAM 2—PATIENT 9

PDX	038.42	Septicemia due to Escherichia coli (E. coli)
DX2	590.10	Acute pyelonephritis, without lesion of renal medullary necrosis
DX3	054.9	Herpes simplex without mention of complication
DX4	V09.0	Infection with microorganisms resistant to penicillins
DX5	305.1	Tobacco use disorder

Notes on Patient 9

038.42 *E coli* septicemia is documented on the culture and sensitivity as well as in the discharge summary. SIRS is not used here because septicemia is documented (versus sepsis) (Brown 2011, 109).

590.10 Acute pyelonephritis is also coded because this is where the septicemia began. Do not code the organism (*Coding Clinic* 4th Quarter 1988). It is already reflected in the septicemia code (Brown 2011, 217).

054.9 Herpes simplex is documented on the 9/8 progress notes and is treated (Brown 2011, chapter 10).

305.1 Tobacco abuse is treated and documented in the progress notes, H & P and D/C summary. This code does not require a fifth digit (HHS 2010, Tabular Index; Brown 2011, chapter 12).

V09.0 The organism is specified to be resistant to in the discharge summary and therefore designate that in the coding (Brown 2011, 113).

Note: The pyelogram performed on 9/8 is not coded because it is an unspecified pyelogram (refer to the Coding Guidelines (in the Introduction of this book). A pyelogram is coded only if it is code 87.74 or 87.76 (Retrogrades, urinary systems).

Points of Interest on Patient 9

1. This case illustrates how an infection can begin in one organ system and then become systemic. This is why the same organism is in the urinary tract and the blood. As stated earlier, code both disorders (septicemia and pyelonephritis).
2. The organism causing the infection is resistant to Penicillin and Ampicillin. Only code resistance to a drug if the resistance is documented by the practitioner in the record. Do not code from the laboratory reports alone.

EXAM 2—PATIENT 10

PDX	276.51	Dehydration
DX2	787.91	Diarrhea
DX3	E936.4	Adverse effect, anti-Parkinsonism drugs
DX4	332.0	Paralysis agitans (Parkinsonism or Parkinson's disease)
DX5	530.81	Esophageal reflux
DX6	403.91	Hypertensive chronic kidney disease, unspecified
DX7	428.0	Congestive heart failure, unspecified
DX8	585.5	Chronic kidney disease, stage V

Notes on Patient 10

276.51 Dehydration is documented in the H & P and discharge summary and is the focus of treatment. Diarrhea and dehydration are both treated. Sequence 276.51 first because this condition is the focus of treatment (*Coding Clinic* 2nd Quarter 1988, 9; Brown 2011, 29).

787.91 Diarrhea due to Sinemet (*Coding Clinic* 3rd Quarter 1995, 10; Brown 2011, 435).

E936.4 Adverse reaction to Sinemet (Brown 2011, 437–438).

332.0 Parkinson's disease is documented in the discharge summary (Brown 2011, 166).

530.81 Esophageal reflux is documented in the discharge summary (Brown 2011, 208–210).

428.0 Documented in the medical record and treated. Based on UHDDS criteria, the CHF is evaluated and monitored. Patient is also receiving medication, and CHF is a chronic condition. For all these reasons, this condition should be coded (Brown 2011, 339–340).

403.91; 585.5 Both are documented in the discharge summary. *ICD-9-CM Official Guidelines for Coding and Reporting* (HHS 2010, Section I, C, 7, a) require both the combination hypertension code and chronic kidney disease code (Brown 2011, chapter 24).

Points of Interest on Patient 10

1. The crux of coding this case revolves around the adverse reaction to Sinemet. This is somewhat challenging because Sinemet is not in the *ICD-9-CM Official Guidelines for Coding and Reporting.* It is, however, a common anti-Parkinson's drug. An experienced coder should know this drug is associated with this disease and subsequently understand how to code an adverse effect.

2. Both the dehydration and diarrhea (the adverse effect) are treated and the two diagnoses do not appear to equally meet the definition of principal diagnosis because the dehydration is the focus of treatment. Because of this the dehydration is sequenced first.

EXAM 2—PATIENT 11

PDX	287.31	Immune thrombocytopenic purpura (ITP)
DX2	571.2	Alcoholic cirrhosis of liver
DX3	250.01	Diabetes mellitus without mention of complication, type 1 [juvenile type], not stated as uncontrolled
DX4	303.93	Other and unspecified alcohol dependence, in remission
DX5	414.00	Coronary atherosclerosis of unspecified type of vessel, native or graft
DX6	518.5	Pulmonary insufficiency following trauma and surgery
DX7	272.4	Other and unspecified hyperlipidemia
DX8	401.9	Essential hypertension, unspecified
DX9	V45.81	Aortocoronary bypass status
DX10	V12.54	Personal history of transient ischemic attack (TIA), and cerebral infarction without residual deficits
PP1	41.5	Total splenectomy
PR2	96.71	Continuous invasive mechanical ventilation for less than 96 consecutive hours
PR3	96.04	Insertion of endotracheal tube

Notes on Patient 11

287.31	Idiopathic thrombocytopenic purpura is documented in the H & P and discharge summary (Brown 2011, chapter 13).
571.2, 303.93	Cirrhosis of the liver is diagnosed with this condition in association with the alcohol use in the progress notes on 6/24. The fifth digit of "3" was used because the patient stopped the alcohol one month before admission (Brown 2011, chapter 12).
250.01, 414.00	These chronic conditions should be coded as it meets the UHDDS criteria for an "other diagnosis" (HHS 2010 Section III, 89).
518.5	Postoperative respiratory distress is documented in the 6/24 progress notes (Brown 2011, chapter 15).
272.4, 401.9	Chronic conditions that are being treated and therefore meet the UHDDS criteria as "other" diagnoses.
V45.81,	The history of these cardiovascular conditions likely contributes to the overall morbidity V12.54 of this patient and must be considered as part of the patient's monitoring during the admission (Brown 2011, chapter 8).
41.5	Splenectomy documented on the operative report (Brown 2011, chapter 7).
96.04; 96.71	These conditions are coded as they are treating the postoperative respiratory failure based on documentation on 6/24 (Brown 2011, 194).

Points of Interest on Patient 11

1. As is evident from the documentation, this case provides practice coding respiratory distress following surgery.
2. This case also provides the opportunity to code alcoholism and a related physical condition.
3. According to the exam coding instructions (in the Introduction of this book), 99.05 transfusion platelet and 99.04 transfusion of PRBC are not coded as per test specifications.

EXAM 2—PATIENT 12

PDX	428.0	Congestive heart failure, unspecified
DX2	397.0	Diseases of tricuspid valve
DX3	250.01	Diabetes mellitus without mention of complication, type 1 [juvenile type], not stated as uncontrolled
DX4	110.1	Dermatophytosis of nail
DX5	703.8	Diseases of nail, hypertrophy
DX6	401.9	Essential hypertension, unspecified
DX7	305.1	Tobacco use disorder
PP1	86.27	Debridement of nail, nailbed, or nail fold
PR2	86.27	Debridement of nail, nailbed, or nail fold

Notes on Patient 12

428.0 The patient is admitted with CHF as documented on the H & P and discharge summary. Even though the patient also has tricuspid valve insufficiency, use the 428.0 because, there is no documentation the CHF is rheumatic (*Coding Clinic* 2nd Quarter 2000, 16–17; Brown 2011, 339–340).

397.0 Tricuspid insufficiency is documented on the discharge summary and H & P (Brown 2011, 330–331).

250.01 Diabetes mellitus type 1 is documented on the discharge summary and H & P. The V code is not used because type 1 diabetes requires insulin (Brown 2011, 121–123; *Coding Clinic* 4th Quarter 2004, 55).

110.1 Mycotic nails (703.8), Hypertrophic nails (401.9), Hypertension (305.1), and tobacco abuse are all documented in the medical record and meet the UHDDS definition (HHS, 2010, Section III, 89). 305.1 does not require a fifth digit (HHS 2010, Tabular Index).

86.27 Debridement of nails performed as per the progress notes and the consult sheet. As per the exam coding instructions (in the Introduction of this book), "Code all procedures that fall within the code range 00.01–86.99, but do not code 57.94 (Foley catheter)." This is coded twice because it is a bilateral debridement.

Points of Interest on Patient 12

1. This case provides an example of the coding rules for coding congestive heart failure with a heart valve disorder (*Coding Clinic* 2nd Quarter 2000, 16–17).
2. The documentation is interesting because the only place the procedure is documented is in the consultation. This is a practice in some healthcare facilities and illustrates the need to review every document in the record in order to code accurately.

EXAM 2—PATIENT 13

PDX	634.11	Spontaneous abortion complicated by delayed or excessive hemorrhage, incomplete
DX2	649.03	Tobacco use disorder complicating pregnancy, childbirth, or the puerperium, antepartum condition or complication
DX3	648.43	Other current conditions in the mother complicating pregnancy, mental disorders, antepartum complication
DX4	311	Depressive disorder, not elsewhere classified
DX5	305.01	Alcohol abuse, continuous
PP1	69.02	Dilatation and curettage following delivery or abortion

Notes on Patient 13

634.11 This is a case of an incomplete spontaneous abortion. This is evidenced by the pathology report. The patient has documented heavy bleeding that has resulted in anemia. Therefore, use the fourth digit of "1" and a fifth digit of "1" (Brown 2011, 278–279).

649.03 Tobacco abuse is also documented and treated. The pregnancy (649.03) code is specific to tobacco abuse and because of this, only use one code (Brown 2011, 277, 296).

69.02 The patient underwent a D & C following spontaneous abortion (Brown 2011, 294).

648.43, 311, 305.01 These conditions are coded to add further specificity. Alcohol abuse is treated and relevant to the case. The physician documented the patient had "alcohol abuse", even though clinically the patient may have alcoholism. Therefore, alcohol abuse, the diagnosis that is documented, is the one that is coded (*Coding Clinic* 2nd Quarter 1998, 13–14). The fifth digit of "3" is used as the patient did not deliver and the conditions were antepartum (Brown 2011, 277).

Points of Interest on Patient 13

1. This case illustrates the difference between coding an incomplete spontaneous abortion and a complication of abortion. In the documentation of the record, the patient had a D & C to complete the spontaneous abortion. A coder might think this should be coded with a code from the 639 category. However, if there are products of conception or other material from the pregnancy retained in the uterus at the time of readmission, this indicates the abortion was not completed. Therefore, use the 634 category. If, on the other hand, there was no retained material, use the 639 category (complication of spontaneous abortion).

2. Spontaneous abortion and miscarriage are used interchangeably in *ICD-9-CM Official Guidelines for Coding and Reporting.*

CCS References

References

American College of Radiology (ACR) and the Radiological Society of North America (RSNA). 2010 (March). CT Colonography: http://www.radiologyinfo.org/en/info.cfm?pg=ct_colo.

American Health Information Management Association. 2008. Code of Ethics and the Standards of Ethical Coding. http://www.ahima.org/about/ethics.asp. Chicago: AHIMA.

American Health Information Management Association AHIMA's Compliance Task Force. 1999 (Jan.). Practice Brief: Seven Steps to Corporate Compliance. *Journal of AHIMA*. Chicago: AHIMA.

American Health Information Management Association. 2010. *Pocket Glossary of Health Information Management and Technology,* Second Edition. Chicago: AHIMA.

American Health Information Management Association. 2008 (Oct.). Practice Brief: Managing an effective query process. *Journal of AHIMA* 79(10): 83–88.

American Hospital Association. 1984, 1987–1990, 1992, 1993, 1995, 1997, 1998, 2000, 2001, 2002, 2004–2010. Coding Clinic for ICD-9-CM. Chicago: AHA Services. *(Refer to the answer key for specifics.)*

American Medical Association. 2011. *CPT Professional Edition.* Chicago: AMA.

American Medical Association. 1995, 1996, 1999, 2000, 2001, 2003, 2005, 2008, 2009, 2010. *CPT Assistant.* Chicago: AMA. *(Refer to the answer key for specifics.)*

American Medical Association. CPT Changes Insider's View. 2006, 2009, 2010, 2011. Chicago: AMA. *(Refer to the answer key for specifics.)*

America Pregnancy Association (APA). 2007. Cephalopelvic disproportion (CPD): www.americanpregnancy.org/labornbirth/cephalopelvicdisproportion.html.

Bowman, Sue. 2007. *Health Information Management Compliance Guidelines for Preventing Fraud and Abuse,* Fourth Edition. Chicago: AHIMA.

Brodnik, Melanie, McCain, Mary, Rinehart-Thompson, Laurie, and Rebecca Reynolds. 2009. *Fundamentals of Law for Health Informatics and Health Information Management.* Chicago: AHIMA.

Brown, Faye (author) and Nelly Leon-Chisen (editor). 2011. *ICD-9-CM Coding Handbook with Answers,* Revised Edition. Chicago: AHA Services.

Centers for Medicare and Medicaid Services (CMS). 2010. http://www.cms.gov/AcuteInpatientPPS/FFD/ItemDetail.asp?ItemID=CMS1230516 (Search for DRG relative weights.)

Casto, Anne B. and Elizabeth Layman. 2011. *Principles of Healthcare Reimbursement, Third Edition.* Chicago: AHIMA.

Clark, Andrea. 2009 (March). "Key Issues in the 2009 OPPS Final Rule" *Journal of AHIMA* 80(3):72–73.

Center for Medicare and Medicaid (CMS) Division of Institutional Claims Processing. 2008. "Definition and Uses of Health Insurance Prospective Payment System Codes (HIPPS Codes). https://www.cms.gov/ProspMedicareFeeSvcPmtGen/downloads/hippsusesv4.pdf.

Davis, Nadinia and Melissa LaCour. 2007. *Health Information Technology.* Philadelphia: Saunders.

DeVault, Kathy. 2010. CPT Coding Updates. *Journal of AHIMA* 81(2):62–63, 66. Chicago: AHIMA.

Dorland's Medical Dictionary, 27th ed. 2000. Baltimore: Lippincott, Williams and Wilkins.

Garrett, Gail S. 2009. *Present on Admission,* Second Edition. Chicago: AHIMA.

Hazelwood, Anita C., and Carol A. Venable. 2011. *ICD-9-CM Diagnostic Coding and Reimbursement for Physician Services.* Chicago: AHIMA.

Innovative Resources for Payers (IRP). 2007. Grouper: www.irp.com.

Johns, Merida (volume editor). 2011. *Health Information Management Technology,* Third Edition. Chicago: AHIMA.

Kuehn, Lynn. 2011. *Procedural Coding and Reimbursement for Physician Services: Applying Current Procedural Terminology and HCPCS.* Chicago: AHIMA.

LaTour, Kathleen and Shirley Eichenwald Maki (volume editors) 2010. *Health Information Management: Concepts, Principles, and Practice,* Third Edition. Chicago: AHIMA.

Lovaasen, K.R. and Schwerdtfeger, J. 2011. *ICD-9-CM Coding: Theory and Practice,* Second Edition. Health Sciences Division: Elsevier.

Medicare Grouper. 2010. Version 28-10/10.

Schraffenberger, Lou Ann. 2010. *Basic ICD-9-CM Coding.* Chicago: AHIMA.

Schraffenberger, Lou Ann. 2007. *Effective Management of Coding Services.* Chicago: AHIMA.

Scott, Karen S. 2009. *Coding and Reimbursement for Hospital Inpatient Services,* Second Edition. Chicago: AHIMA.

Smith, Gail I. 2011. *Basic Current Procedural Terminology and HCPCS Coding,* 2011. Chicago: AHIMA.

US Department of Health and Human Services (HHS). 2010. International Classification of Diseases, Ninth Revision, Clinical Modification (ICD-9_CM). http://www.cdc.gov/nchs/data/icd9/icdguide10.pdf.

US Department of Health and Human Services. 2003 (Jan. 1). Medicare Conditions of Participation: Medical Staff: http://www.access.gpo.gov/nara/cfr/waisidx_03/42cfr482_03.html.

Additional Resources

AHIMA Communities of Practice (CoP): http://cop.ahima.org

AHIMA Certification: www.ahima.org/certification

ICD-9-CM Coding

Clinical Coding Workout: Practice Exercises for Skill Development, (with Answers) 2011. Chicago: AHIMA.

HCPCS and CPT Coding

Principles of CPT Coding. Chicago: American Medical Association.

http://www.cms.gov/HCPCSReleaseCodeSets/ANHCPCS/list.asp#TopOfPage (Search for FY 11)2011_CCS_References.docx

Regulatory Guidelines, Data Quality, and Compliance

Books

Kennedy, James S. 2008. *Severity DRGs and Reimbursement:* An MS-DRG Primer. Chicago: AHIMA.

2011 DRG Desk Reference. 2011. Ingenix.

Websites

APCs and status indicators (for 2011): https://www.cms.gov/HospitalOutpatientPPS/ (Search for *addendum B.*)

Common medications and associated diseases: www.rxlist.com

Decision trees, stress management, and other topics: http://www.mindtools.com/dectree.html. *(Note: Decision trees form the basis of DRG trees, which are found on the national exam. It is important to review this website.)*

DRG grouper (free): irp.com *(Disclaimer: This software application may contain errors and is not endorsed or developed by the author or AHIMA.)*

MS-DRG weights for 2011: https://www.cms.gov/AcuteInpatientPPS/FFD/list.asp#TopOfPage (Search for FY 2011 DRG weights.)

Present on admission information: http://www.cms.hhs.gov/HospitalAcqCond/01_Overview.asp

Documentation, Information and Communication Technologies and Privacy, Confidentiality, Legal, and Ethical Issues

Thomason, Mary C. 2008. *HIPAA by Example*. Chicago: AHIMA.

Amatayakul, Margret K. 2009. *Electronic Health Records: A Practical Guide for Professionals and Organizations,* Fourth Edition. Chicago: AHIMA.